Ethical Issues
in Mental Health

Edited by
Philip J. Barker PhD

Clinical Nurse Consultant
Honorary Lecturer
University of Dundee
UK

and

Steve Baldwin PhD

Consultant Psychologist
Visiting Research Fellow
Polytechnic South West
Plymouth
UK

CHAPMAN & HALL
London · Glasgow · New York · Tokyo · Melbourne · Madras

362.2

Published by Chapman & Hall, 2-6 Boundary Row, London SE1 8HN

Chapman & Hall, 2-6 Boundary Row, London SE1 8HN, UK

Blackie Academic & Professional, Wester Cleddens Road,
Bishopbriggs, Glasgow G64 2NZ, UK

Chapman & Hall, 29 West 35th Street, New York NY10001, USA

Chapman & Hall Japan, Thomson Publishing Japan, Hirakawacho
Nemoto Building, 6F, 1-7-11 Hirakawa-cho, Chiyoda-ku, Tokyo 102,
Japan

Chapman & Hall Australia, Thomas Nelson Australia, 102 Dodds
Street, South Melbourne, Victoria 3205, Australia

Chapman & Hall India, R. Seshadri, 32 Second Main Road, CIT East,
Madras 600 035, India

First edition 1991
Reprinted 1992

© 1991 Chapman & Hall

Phototypeset in 10/12pt Palatino by Intype, London
Printed in Great Britain by Page Bros (Norwich) Ltd

ISBN 0 412 32950 6

A catalogue record for this book is available from the British Library

Library of Congress Cataloging-in-Publication data available

Contents

Contributors

Jaqueline Atkinson is Lecturer in the Department of Community Medicine, University of Glasgow

Phil Barker is Clinical Nurse Consultant at the Mental Health Unit, Tayside Health Board, and Honorary Lecturer, University of Dundee

Steve Baldwin is Consultant Psychologist, Neighbourhoods Network, TACADE, Salford: Visiting Research Fellow, Department of Psychology, Polytechnic South West

Christine Barrowclough was Principal Clinical Psychologist at District Psychology Department, Prestwich Hospital, Manchester

David Brandon is Psychotherapist, Freelance Trainer and Social Worker, TAO, 36 Victoria Parade, Ashton, Preston

Liam Clarke is Nurse Teacher (Psychiatry), Sussex Downs School of Nursing, Hellingly Hospital, Hailsham

Chris Cullen is Scottish Society for Mental Handicap (SSMH), Chair of Learning Difficulties at the University of St Andrews

Philip Darbyshire is Lecturer at the Department of Nursing, Glasgow College

Tony Ellis is Professor of Philosophy at Virginia Commonwealth University, USA, and was previously the Co-founder of the Centre for Philosophy and Public Affairs at University of St Andrews

Ian Fleming is Principal Clinical Psychologist at Swinton Hospital, Manchester

Ian Stewart is a retired Consultant Psychiatrist: he was Consultant in Forensic Psychiatry at Rampton Special Hospital (1978–81) and Consultant Psychotherapist at Castel Hospital, Guernsey (1976–78)

Martin Ward is Psychiatric Nurse Tutor at Hellesdon Hospital, Norwich

Acknowledgements

The editors would like to acknowledge the support of Christine Birdsall in promoting the original idea of the book. The invaluable assistance of Bette Harris and Carol Miller, in the production of the manuscript, is also warmly acknowledged.

Preface

Why write another book on ethics?

As practitioners we are involved both in the design and delivery of services to people with mental health problems. In common with all other professionals, our work has led to the experience of ethical dilemmas: typically, these have involved major confrontations, either with our colleagues or our consciences.

This book, however, is not limited to a discussion of such major themes. Rather, we have tried to use a broader canvas: ethics, in our view, is really about the judgement of right and wrong in ordinary, everyday life. Ethics are highly personal: we fashion our own personal code from our experience of others, and from the 'tests' which bring meaning to our lives. Such experiences shape our individual values.

We bring these codes and values to our work. We are not always aware of their influence in our dealings with people. Although we may not always be aware of it, all our actions pose an ethical question. Given that our work involves us in helping others to live ordinary, satisfying lives, this challenge heightens the intensity of our ethical dilemmas. This is most evident where our personal code conflicts with the implicit code of the health setting.

This book is fundamentally about this axis of ethics: do people follow a personal code, or do they adhere to implicit codes? We also wish to examine the extent to which personal codes influence those of other professionals. At present, professional codes reflect different priorities, fail to share a common ground and may, in the final analysis, be self-protecting rather than liberating.

One aim of this book is to examine the difficulties which people experience, either in providing or receiving mental health services. In selecting the contributors we wished to represent a broad spectrum of practitioners who could comment on their own field of interest, primarily from the view of the person in need of mental health services. In our view any service which is not focused, unashamedly, on the person risks losing the person. Clearly, services exist which not only 'lose' people, but systematically destroy them in the process. In our consideration of ethics we should remember that every day 'wrongs' occur in most systems: this is the nub of the ethical enquiry.

Throughout this book there is an acknowledgement that no easy answers exist to what are complex themes. In our conclusion we offer some recommendations: these are not comprehensive, but may provide the starting point for further discussion. We hope you will join us in this debate.

Phil Barker and Steve Baldwin
Newport-on-Tay

Foreword

Traditional wisdom dictates that one's definition of a human problem determines one's response to that problem. The focus of this book admirably defines and responds to the ethical issues around the well-being of 'persons in care for mental health problems associated with living'. The human dignity of persons with mental health problems or with varying degrees of mental retardation is espoused as a consistent theme by the editors and developed by the contributors in the wide-ranging topics addressed by this work. 'Persons in care' is not a semantic device used in place of the more traditional term 'patient' or the more progressive term 'client' in describing our fellow citizens in need of care in a variety of mental health care settings. The term is chosen to avoid the dehumanization of labelling and to provide vision for the wider perspective of human potential central to this work.

The ethical stance of the work is both commendable and engaging. It avoids pure philosophical inquiry of a purely theoretical genre which is unrelated to the everyday issues involved in the care of persons with mental health problems. It, likewise, shuns a purely subjective approach which could consist of an array of well-meaning opinion or conjecture, lacking the benefit of any ethical analysis. The work is firmly grounded in the day-to-day realities of the human relationships between professionals and persons in care as the principles of self-determination, paternalism and fairness determine the human dimensions of day-to-day decision making. The real power of this work and its unique contribution is to be found in the humane balance of accepted ethical theory and principle in their application to clinical practice within the context of real life, individual and institutional. The values and ideas of the professional care-givers are critically examined in their effect on the lives of those for whom they care.

The reality of the ethical problems, resulting from the conflict between institutional policy and the ethical standards of mental health care professionals, are excellently treated. The turf wars between the various professionals, within the hierarchical structure which characterizes the delivery of mental health care in almost every country, are presented in an open and honest fashion. The tone of the many contributions is mercifully free from the turf-guarding and fingerpointing which characterizes much of the writing in this arena. Rather than being a polemic directed against this status quo, this work proposes and defines a unified and practical ethical agenda which has the ability to unite policy makers, institutional leaders and health care professionals for many disciplines around 'persons in care' centred issues of advocacy, access, assessment, goals, evaluation and the accountability.

The absence of adequate teaching around ethical issues in the professional training of mental healthcare professionals is well established. The inability of professionals to identify ethical issues as the impact on their work and morale is traced to this. An ability to engage in meaningful dialogue at the societal level, and especially across the professions and at all levels of institutional policy making is seen as enhancing the quality of life for care-givers and those receiving care. A preoccupation with legal requirements and with procedural guidelines, and an appeal to such as the ultimate arbiters of morality, is seen as detrimental to the more humane, soul-searching inquiry prompted by ethical reflection. Liam Clark, one of the contributing authors, aptly comments: 'Law respects neither justice nor philosophy, only precision'.

The themes and discussions embodied in this work are of universal application. They address the ethical issues involved in mental health work in their significance not only for the United Kingdom but also for the European community and the United States as well. An impressive, up-to-date and significant body of international reference materials supports the arguments and themes presented. This is an outstanding feature of the work.

Writing the foreword to this excellent and timely addition to the dialogue around ethical issues within the mental field is a distinct honour and a labour of love. Professionals from many disciplines will be enlightened as they are challenged by the contents of this work. It promises to be an excellent teaching resource for a variety of professional settings. The compelling arguments of this work, favouring sweeping changes in the mental healthcare delivery system, can be used by citizens dedicated to promoting the welfare of persons with mental health problems. Cogent ethical persuasion can add bite and decisiveness to their efforts.

Above all, this work sensitizes all of us to the human needs of Joe, a person 'in care' who is described in the vignette 'Home and Away' at the conclusion of the book. Joe is 'a quiet man leading a quiet life; he eases himself effortlessly from the institutional to everyday life and back again, attracting no special attention'. He gardens, he bowls, he attends and enjoys soccer games at home and away; he is fully involved in the life of his community. Well-meaning persons remove him from his familiar surroundings to a more 'humane residential setting in a quiet seaside town'. He is far from his familiar haunts and removed from his productive way of life. There is no more football, no more gardening, but there is a 'life which becomes quieter than ever'. Joe's story eloquently captures the high moral tone of this work.

   The ultimate challenge of this work is enshrined in Joe's story. Our task is to provide the most humane environment for the Joes of our world, wherever they live. The editors and contributors have developed an inspiring moral context to frame our response.

Professor Thomas F. McGovern
Director, Bioethics Program
Department of Psychiatry
Texas Tech University Health Sciences Center
Lubbock Texas USA

Part One

Chapter One

User power

DAVID BRANDON

EDITORS' INTRODUCTION

People for whom services are designed and presented should always be in the forefront of our thinking. People are the primary consideration: what are their needs; what do they want; how do professionals, and people, together achieve this?

It has been acknowledged, at least since Goffman's pioneering work, that institutions often work against the best interests of those in their care. People who experience problems of living need special provisions: services which acknowledge how such people are similar to, as well as different from, the rest of society. Services for people with special needs, whether offered in traditional 'institutions' or in their modern equivalent, have tended to emphasize the 'different' status of people with special needs. In many services the person is overlooked by staff intent on dealing with a diagnostic condition. The person is overshadowed by this label, and may become no more than a number drawn from a classification system.

In this chapter **David Brandon** sets the ethical agenda. Where else should a consideration of ethical behaviour begin but with a consideration of the person as citizen: enjoying the benefits of a democratic society with unalienable rights, and guaranteed participation in any decisions affecting the services he or she needs.

User power

There is one dilemma at the heart of our so-called caring systems, which is rarely analysed, but which has immense moral and political implications. At least notionally, we in the West live in a democracy. Almost every citizen, not actually compulsorily detained in mental hospital or serving a prison sentence, has (in law) the right to vote if he or she chooses. One person — one vote.

The whole concept of being a full citizen in our Western democracies is active and participative. Citizens have the right to speak out, to complain, to be represented, to pursue happiness, to get involved, even to criticize the state publically. There is an inbuilt assumption about more active ordinary citizens — the more power they have, the better. The media repeatedly highlights the immense dangers of popular apathy and alienation. Politicians spend much time explaining issues and events to ordinary voters and, hopefully, listening to how they respond. Traditionally, democracies are contrasted positively with totalitarian countries where, it is claimed, people are not free citizens but lack something called 'human rights', where voting is either nonexistent or a futile exercise. Dictatorship, either by individuals or party caucus, effectively decides for all persons.

One stigmatized group of citizens may have a series of unique obstacles put between them and their vote in the most recent legislation. 'The patient must declare without assistance that he is an informal mental patient, and must give the United Kingdom address where he would be resident if he were not a mental patient.' If a patient cannot give such an address, any UK address (other than a mental hospital) at which he has resided is acceptable. Mental patients residing in a hospital cannot give the address of the institution for voting registration purposes. 'We even place additional barriers on the right to litigation, fearing that they may be vexatious' (Gostin, 1983).

By any standards, our 'caring' systems are essentially totalitarian. Residents, patients and consumers in old peoples homes, hospitals, hostels, day centres have scarcely any say or real influence on either policy or practice in most services. Vital decisions are made commonly by staff, often at senior level, who are not directly accountable to (or even accessible to) ordinary users. Millions of our most vulnerable members live without most of the valued benefits and protections of democracy. They are almost entirely at the mercy of those who 'care' for them. It is extremely difficult to see from what source those service staff get their authority to practice.

An example of a hospital admission will illustrate:

> The nurse took my tablets off me and made a final brisk squiggle on her clip-board. 'There's a list of mealtimes and a washing-up rota on the notice board upstairs' she said. 'Toilets and bathroom down the corridor on the left. If you want a bath ask a nurse for the taps.' It was as simple as that. Ten minutes ago I had been a responsible adult — a senior social worker. Now I was a patient in a psychiatric unit and had to ask for bath taps. It all seemed unreal, like a scene from a play, except I was alone in a room in a psychiatric unit and the play did not end.
>
> (Brandon, 1981)

Or this:

> On arrival at mental hospital to keep my out-patient appointment with the community psychiatric nurse, the doctor refused to have any conversation with me and simply discussed me, in the third person, with a

nurse. I was then instructed that I was to be detained upon section since I was 'high', confronted by two large coloured male nurses and escorted to the ward where I was deprived of my clothes and possessions, and detained despite my protestations.

(Brandon, 1981)

Recently, a consultant psychiatrist instructed the unit sister that none of 'his' patients were to talk to a team authorized to evaluate the hospital facility without his specific permission. The most interesting element in this event may have been the thought they were 'his' patients, almost literally? Or that the ward sister accepted his instructions? The patients were not consulted at all.

From these descriptions, hospital based staff felt that 'their patients' had few rights. They are not citizens any more. They had been transformed into 'patients' so quite a different set of rules was applied. Valued human rights, along with their clothing, freedom to choose with whom they talked, personal privacy, freedom of movement, basic dignity and individuality were stripped away, often without any explanation. To add insult to injury, it was claimed that these rights were stripped away for 'their own good.'

It would be naive to assume that such practices are confined to the psychiatric sector. An account of life in a long stay hospital by a man with a mental handicap illustrates this:

Being in the institution was bad. I got tied up and locked up. I didn't have any clothes of my own, and no privacy. We got beat at times but that wasn't the worst. The real pain came from being always being in a group. I was never a person. I was part of a group to eat, sleep and everything. As a kid I couldn't figure out who I was. I was part of a group. I was sad.

(Ryan and Thomas, 1980)

In a mental handicap hostel study (Brandon and Ridley, 1985), excellent service philosophies were found stressing the importance of freedom, individual choices and participation. They had no discernable impact on reality however. The 26 residents had hardly any control over their own lives, despite excellent philosophical principles. They wanted to live in ordinary housing and have a proper job with real wages. They got a mini-institution and £4.00 a week at a local Adult Training Centre.

These experiences are widespread, in various forms and degrees, in most human services. It is unimaginable that ordinary hotels could be run along these lines. Customers would choose to go elsewhere and hotels would go bankrupt. Real choices do not exist in most of the public sector. Most professionals have an effective monopoly.

Most present practice differs substantially from what is envisioned by some professionals as a good standard. Ramon (1985) observes: 'The drugging of the majority of those who express unhappiness can be seen as a major exercise of social containment of dissatisfaction. But let us not forget that it also represents a major deviation from the stated value preferences of every one of the involved professional group.'

Social workers, doctors, psychologists and nurses assimilate a set of values during training, and then often adhere to quite another (inferior) set after qualification. Professional culture is much more powerful than any training. There are thousands of studies on the institutionalization of consumers, but relatively few on the important topic of staff institutionalization. Young staff newcomers quickly get brutalized into institutionally acceptable ways of behaving.

A man in his thirties had been working in the mental handicap service for three weeks. After years of unemployment himself, he expressed surprise at how lazy some people with mental handicaps were; 'It's the devil to get them up early in the morning.' He had forgotten about his own timekeeping and general industry when he was not being paid. He was already being institutionalized into embarrassing concepts such as 'laziness' which ignored the context in which people were living.

Freedom and personal choice are highly valued in theory but, in practice, however desirable, those general principles are often highly circumscribed. For example in research into 175 local authority homes for elderly people, Booth (1985) quotes a senior staff member saying: 'Everyone can stay up for as long as they want, including the handicapped once they are undressed.' Booth discovered that: 'very few homes (only 18%) offered residents a choice of main dishes on the menu for the main meal. Fewer than half of the homes (44%) allowed the residents to choose their own bathtimes. In the remainder it was the staff who decided who was to bath and when' (Booth, 1985).

In the North West of England study, 'Consumers as Colleagues', two services were assessed a local authority psychiatric hostel, and a psychiatric hospital long stay ward, for evidence of democracy (Brandon and Brandon, 1987).

Although these services were part of two quite different cultures (NHS and local authority) there was little involvement by consumers in the running of either service. Neither hostel nor ward had consumers on management bodies; neither involved them in selection of staff; neither permitted access to case files or case conferences where they were discussed. They were being 'done to' rather than worked with — in a very colonial manner. One hospital patient said: 'Being here is like being in the forces'.

Studies of participation in old people's homes (for example Booth, 1985), have uncovered a very similar picture. Staff and residents met regularly together formally to discuss common affairs in less than a third (29%) of the homes. Just under half (46%) held regular staff meetings, but a quarter of the homes had no regular meetings involving staff or residents. By not having some formal mechanism for participation, residents were being denied the opportunity of expressing their collective opinions on the running of the home; old people were thus deprived of full citizenship. Staff were conventionally and regularly behaving to users in ways which they would find totally unacceptable were they on the receiving end, thus practising a form of social apartheid.

Key ethical and political questions arise from this central dilemma — some people are having some or all of their citizenship stripped away by human services, whilst still living inside a 'democracy'. How can this take place? If the services are not primarily about what professionals say they are about (serving and caring for consumers) then what really drives them? If professionals and their employing agencies are not meaningfully accountable to service consumers, then to whom, if anyone, are they accountable?

Service staff managers justify this totalitarian situation through a fog of rationalizations. 'They don't want to be bothered with all that'. 'We are trained professionals — we really know what is best for them'. 'We've always run services like that'. 'They're mentally ill . . . handicapped . . . old . . . They don't understand how to make real choices'. Such justifications are simply signs of powerful underlying currents. The massive effect of the institution on the individual's behaviour has been lost.

These consumers are entering situations and adopting roles which, traditionally are socially devalued. Wolfensberger (1972) describes the whole process whereby some people, no longer seen as contributing economically or socially, become ensnared in a vicious spiral in which they are perceived as losing value in the eyes of others, and eventually themselves. They become inadequate, socially stigmatized and chronically deviant. Sick, handicapped and old people are seen by relatively powerful others to be less than fully human — subnormal, (sic), immature, childish, even menacing and threatening. The more chronic the condition, the more the person concerned is devalued. Some areas, particularly 'mental illness' and 'mental handicap' are traditionally highly stigmatized.

Symbols and imagery linked with devalued people are overwhelmingly negative. They help spawn and magnify 'disabilism'. Media images build up an almost entirely negative picture of disabled people — from *Psycho* to Smike in Dickens' *Nicholas Nickleby*. Millions of posters, radio references, TV programmes and banner newspaper headlines try to elicit feelings of fear, disgust, ridicule, superiority, pity and sympathy. Tragic heroes and heroines jostle with monsters and animals. 'Locals petition against home for junkies'; 'Mad axeman slays innocent child'. One poster (UN, 1982) reads: 'Herb Ross will be eight years old for the rest of his life'. This poster shows Herb in the 'perpetual child mode' as if he had no possibility of growing up to be an adult. Many major voluntary organizations like Mencap and Spastics Society capitalize upon advertizing campaigns which devalue the people they are meant to serve. (Wertheimer, 1988).

Example

In the deep shade, at the farther end of the room, a figure ran backwards and forwards. What it was, whether beast or human being, one could not, at first sight, tell. It grovelled, seemingly on all fours: it snatched and growled like some strange wild animal. But it was covered in clothing, and a quantity of dark, grizzled hair wild as a mane, hid its head and face.

The first and 'mad' Mrs Rochester meets the lady who is destined to be the second Mrs Rochester (Charlotte Brontë's *Jane Eyre*). How would you feel about going over and talking to that figure about your favourite country walk or meal?

Even the typically more sober and professional language contributes to the same devaluing process — 'subnormals', 'retardates,' 'schizophrenics', 'the elderly' — as if the disability dominated the whole person. We can see the wheelchair but somehow the person gets lost. A leading expert on mental handicap (Heaton-Ward, 1977) has said: 'The most serious sexual problems are likely to arise in mildly mentally-handicapped women who have a strong sexual drive, but impaired self control.' This is a value-laden, stereotyping, generalization.

Without ordinary rights of full citizens, these devalued people have frequently entered institutions which are 'special' (i.e. segregated, of poor quality), where they are herded together in large dayrooms and dormitories. In such surroundings there may be little respect for personal sexuality, privacy, individuality. In these congregated and segregated settings (homes, particularly long stay hospital, hostels, day centres), their deviancy, terminal condition, physical disability, homelessness (etc.) will become magnified. People sometimes live most of their lives in poverty and institutional humiliation while their dignity is stripped away. Under enormous pressure, they begin to blame themselves. They internalize socially negative processes, and feel they are essentially a burden to others, as having little human use. They begin to blame themselves for this feeling; they let others down and are not 'good enough.'

One major purpose of these services is not to 'care' for people but rather to control them. The primary purpose is to render its users both harmless and marginal, to ensure they exist on the extreme edges of our society with little power, influence or money. 'Psychiatry functions, not indeed as a centrepiece, but as one wing of a nineteenth century strategy of transcribing problems of collective order, social, political and economic, into problems of morality; that sector of the population that cannot be assimilated to society by methods of improvement must be neutralized as a social danger' (Gordon, 1986).

Hospitals are ghettos, which keep large numbers of devalued people apart from the ordinary valued population. The socialization and training of nurses, doctors and other professionals, especially for long-stay institutions, has been primarily directed towards this. 'Smaller armies of professional handlers are paid to identify the human problems, classify and label them in a way that allows them to be packaged and sent out of the public arena to some suitably named 'warehouse' manned by public servants, who indeed serve the public by locking up the bits of human reality that they find unsavoury (Corry, 1986). This army of nurses and doctors functions as gatekeepers, mainly preventing egress to the wider society. Such a process is fundamentally immoral.

The most well know pseudo-patient psychiatric study (Rosenham, 1973) has illustrated some of these wider processes. A psychologist and seven other persons were admitted to 12 hospitals in the USA. They stayed in these hospitals from a few weeks to several months. Their day-to-day behaviour on the ward was seen as symptomatic of various pathological conditions, even though they were behaving 'normally', not simulating any pathological conditions. One person taking notes for the study was described in nursing notes as: 'patient engages in writing behaviour'.

> Never were the staff found to assume that one of themselves or the structure of the hospital had anything to do with a patient's behaviour. One psychiatrist pointed to a group of patients who were sitting outside the cafeteria entrance half an hour before lunchtime. To a group of trainee doctors, he indicated that such behaviour was characteristic of the 'oral-acquisitive' nature of the syndrome. It seemed not to occur to him that there were few things to anticipate in a psychiatric hospital beside eating.
>
> (Rosenhan, 1973)

Rosenhan concluded that mental hospitals were characterized by a rigid hierarchical structure. Staff frequently avoided both verbal and nonverbal contact with patients who had initiated a discussion with them. Patients were made to feel powerless and depersonalized, and treatment relied heavily on psychotropic drugs.

How can conditions be improved for people who are devalued in our society? How can we create a revolution? An examination of devaluing processes is required to fight against racism, sexism and disabilism in all its myriad forms. Personal damage, from years of exposure to disabilist material in training courses should be resolved.

Most of all, it needs to be acknowledged that this is primarily a political struggle. An important task for professionals is to help consumers gain more power and control, both over their lives, and over the running of the services. 'It ought thus be made to mean, at least, that the principal of citizenship is not merely a component in the ideal terms of specification of therapeutic objectives, but a continuous criterion of therapeutic action (Gordon, 1986).

The notion of practical citizenship should involve seven stages: improved information systems; consultation; skilled support in decision making; access to independent representation; helping users to plan services; gradual devolution of decision making; and management by users with help of staff (Brandon, 1987).

Most services are secretive: information is shared grudgingly. The recent Disabled Persons (Services, Consultation and Representation) Act (1986) should encourage the freer flow of information. It does not, however, apply to the NHS. Users need access to relevant written material, attendance at case conferences and access to files.

The long and arduous battle of 'Ann', labelled educationally subnormal, for access to her social service and medical files, illustrates this (Sinclair, 1986).

Information is of very limited value if people are not also consulted. Birmingham Social Services Department asked people with 'mental illness' and 'mental handicap' what they wanted from services (Ritchie *et al.*, 1987). NIMROD, a Cardiff-based mental handicap service has sponsored several consultative exercises where users are asked about the kinds of services they would like (Lowe *et al.*, 1985).

Users will need skilled support in decision-making. Services have been so crushing of initiative that people will require support in deciding for themselves. They need assertiveness training as well as help in self-advocacy. One pioneering Housing Association (Edinvar, Edinburgh), for example, builds self-advocacy into its neighbourhood support schemes (Edinvar, 1987).

To resist those powerful pressures, they will need access to independent representation. One potent form of this is citizen advocacy. 'One-to-one' volunteer systems are developed totally independently of service deliverers, to represent individual consumers (Morris, 1987). Consumers must also be involved in planning services. In Holland, most psychiatric hospitals have a patients' council subsidized by the government. It has a statutory right to advise the hospital authorities on policy matters. Nottingham Patients' Council, established in 1986, had adapted and copied some of the Dutch ideas (Legemaate, 1985). This council, with only former psychiatric patients, has four specific aims: to create more awareness and control by service users; to create user-only meetings in wards, day centres and community mental health centres; to influence the planning and management of mental health services; to educate workers both locally and nationally about the need for user involvement.

People need to experience a gradual devolution of decision-making.

Helping with job appointments is a good and important example. Twenty seven staff appointments in the East Cardiff Mental Handicap Service (ranging from co-ordinators of community mental handicap schemes through to care assistants in community living schemes) have been made, which involved mentally handicapped consumers (Frost, 1986). Their questions have often been direct and penetrating — ranging from: 'How would you find me a job in a pet shop?' to 'Tell us about some of the jobs you have done; how many could be done in centres by people like us?'

The process of devolution eventually may result in effective management by consumers with staff help. For example, Alcoholics Anonymous is run entirely by consumers. There is a national network of locally-based advice and information services run by physically disabled people (Burgess, 1985).

Such a process would begin to restore full citizenship to consumers who have been devalued. These consumers may need money more than they need social workers or nurses. They need resources to play a fuller role in society. Some services are becoming more questioning and flexible.

> The assumption is often made that successful community care depends on the creation of a substantial range of discrete services staffed by a new army of community-based professionals — more social workers, community nurses, paramedical staff, day centres and hostels. While such resources clearly have an important role to play, the recognition must be that the real support for the 80% of the mentally handicapped population who live within the community comes from the infrastructure of the community itself — friends, neighbours and relatives.
>
> (Newman and Cox, 1987)

It will be a long hard struggle to gain power for disabled people. Rachel Hurst, Chair of British Council of Organizations of Disabled People, rightly comments: 'The right to influence decisions affecting their own lives is denied disabled people in Britain today,' (Hurst, 1987). It is part of a gigantic process in which the lives of devalued people have been professionalized and marginalized.

Services are currently a maelstrom of different ideas. Consumerism competes with de-professionalism; quality control with normalization; the advocacy movement with community action (Brandon and Brandon, 1987). There is a move from institutionally-based provision to community care — whatever that means.

All of this will be mainly cosmetic unless there is a complete redistribution of power so that service users have much much more control over their own lives.

REFERENCES

Brandon, D. (1981) *Voices of Experience*. MIND, London.
Brandon, D. (1987) Participation and choice: a worthwhile pilgrimage. *Social Work Today*, **19** (17), 8–9, 21st December.
Brandon, A. and Brandon, D. (1987) *Consumers as Colleagues*, MIND, London.
Brandon, D. and Ridley, J. (1985) *Beginning to Listen*. Campaign for Mental Handicap, London.
Booth, T. (1985) *Home Truths: Old People's Homes and the Outcome of Care*. Gower Medical, London.
Burgess, P. (1985) Keeping the lines open. *Community Care* No. 574, 16–18, 8th August.
Corry, M. (ed.) (1986) Warehousing human problems. In *Institutions: Safety Belts or Strait-jackets? Poverty in Ireland and the role of Four Institutions. Finance, Law, Psychiatry and the Church*. Simon Community, Dublin.
Edinvar (1987) *Building a Housing Foundation for Community Care*. Edinburgh.
Frost, B. (1986) Where selecting staff is a joint effort. *Social Work Today*, **18** (7), 14–15, 13th October.
Gostin, L. (1983) *A Practical Guide to Mental Health Law*. MIND, London.
Heaton-Ward, A. (1977) *Left Behind: A Study of Mental Handicap*. McDonald and Evans, London.
Hurst, R. (1987) Disabled people should influence their own future. *Social Work Today* **18** (21), 30, 26th January.
Legemaate, J. (1985) *Patient's Rights Advocacy: the Dutch model*. Paper given at the World Federation for Mental Health Congress, Brighton.
Lowe, K. *et al.* (1985) *Client's Views: Long Term Evaluation of Services for People With a Mental Handicap in Cardiff*. Applied Research Unit: Mental Handicap in Wales, Cardiff.
Miller, P. and Rose, N. (1986) *The Power of Psychiatry*. Polity Press, New York.
Morris, P. (1987) Making the right match. *Community Living* **12** (2), 14–15.
Newman, T. and Cox, S. (1987) Your flexible friend: South Glamorgan's Flexicare service. *Social Work Today* **18** (26), 14–15, 2nd March.
Ramon, S. (1985) *Psychiatry in Britain — meaning & policy*. Croom Helm, London.
Ritchie, J. *et al.* (1987) Community care needs: the perspective of people with mental illness. *Social and Community Planning Research*.
Rosenhan, D. L. (1973) On being sane in insane places. *Science*, **179**, 250–58.
Ryan, J. and Thomas, F. (1980) *The Politics of Mental Handicap*. Pelican, Harmondsworth.
Sinclair, L. (1986) A plea for access to personal files. *Social Work Today*, **18** (12), 24, 17th November.
United Nations (1982) *Improving Communications about People with Disabilities*. UN, Basle.
Wolfensberger, W. (1972) *Normalization*. National Institute for Mental Retardation, Toronto.

Chapter Two

The nature of morality

TONY ELLIS

EDITORS' INTRODUCTION

All ethical issues ultimately involve consideration of what is 'right' and 'wrong'. Ethics are about ordinary everyday actions, as well as the higher consideration of their value. No service can be evaluated, therefore, without considering what it 'means' to both the person in receipt of the service, and the person delivering the service.

The morality of our actions, what is 'right' or 'wrong', can be confused by reference to other rules which have the potential to restrict the behaviour of individuals within any society. All professionals reading this book will be bound by such rules: codes of conduct, conventions for the practice of professional behaviour. To what extent are such conventions moral in character? All readers, whether professionals or not, will be bound by other 'rules', perhaps less explicitly defined: personal values, religious convictions, and a wide range of social or cultural norms. These are the conventions which provide comfort, or perhaps discomfort, to the individual reader.

In this chapter, **Tony Ellis** considers the fundamental concerns which support the ethical debate. What do cultural conventions, laws, legislation, professional codes of conduct and religious beliefs have in common; and in what way do they differ. What is the nature of morality?

The nature of morality

What is morality? The question is ambiguous and clarity is required. That there is wide and deep disagreement about what is morally right and wrong is all too evident in the field of general medicine. In a wider context differences about morality are even more radical. People differ fundamentally, not only about what is morally right and wrong, but also about the very nature of morality.

An analogy may make this clearer. Imagine, for a moment, that someone asks: 'What is the law?' This could indicate two entirely different questions. The questioner might want to know, roughly, which particular courses of action were legally prohibited, and which were legally permitted. But he or she might have in mind a more abstract question, and might simply want to understand the nature of any legal system; to find the answer without finding out what is legal or illegal in any jurisdiction. The answer to such a question is far from simple, but it would look something like this. The law is a system of rules, enforced in a given society, with the intention of securing that the society is run in some desired way.

Leaving aside the question of which things are right and wrong, what does it mean for something to be morally right or wrong at all? What makes a 'system of rules' a moral system? What makes an ideal a moral ideal? When are praise and blame, moral praise and blame? After all, there are all sorts of rules that are not moral rules (the rules of addition and subtraction, or the rules of cricket, for example). There are ideals that have nothing to do with morality (someone might set themselves the ideal of climbing Mount Everest without oxygen cylinders); and when cold weather is blamed for burst pipes, this has nothing to do with morality.

This analogy with law breaks down at a crucial point. The definition of morality as a kind of law is roughly on the right lines. But it is not straightforward. There is very general, radical dispute about whether a particular reason for taking some course of action is to count as a moral reason, or whether a particular obligation is to count as a moral obligation. This is often thought to be an aspect of the break-up of an adherence to a traditional, shared morality, and is one major cause of current moral perplexities.

It is very hard, therefore, to give any account of the nature of morality which would be generally accepted by modern philosophers. The most that can be done is to give a broad characterization which is as little controversial as possible, and to give some idea of what, to be more precise, are the various ways in which morality may be considered.

MORALITY AND NORMS

Morality is normative. It lays down norms of behaviour; or, in more familiar language, it tells us how to behave. Some people would go further, and say that it is a normative system. This might already be going too far, however, since it suggests that moral principles must have a systematic set of interrelationships, which most people's moral principles do not (on the surface) display. But to say that morality is normative is not to say very much. There are many norms that we follow, which no one would call moral. Comparison of moral norms with other sets of non-moral norms may be useful starting points.

Think, first, of etiquette. The rules of etiquette tell people how to behave at the dinner table and how to address a bishop. Apparently, one ought to eat soup from the side of one's spoon; and when drinking tea from a china cup, one's little finger should stick out at an angle from the rest of one's fingers. Morality is, generally, like this. It tells people how to behave; one ought not to murder, steal and lie. It is a set of norms.

The rules of morality however are different from the rules of etiquette. Imagine that someone at the dinner table eats their soup from the front of their spoon instead of the side. Someone may think this not a pretty sight, but it is not immoral. Why is that?

It just doesn't seem serious enough to be a matter of morality. It must matter to people, in some way, that their fellow guests eat in one way rather than another, though it hardly seems to matter enough to be regarded as a matter of morality. But this does not get to the heart of the matter. After all, morality comes in many degrees of seriousness. If somebody tells a small lie to 'save their face', although this might diminish them morally, few people would think it very serious. The heart of the difference is that there need be no reasons justifying a rule of etiquette. There will always be a reason why some rules of etiquette have evolved (or were created). In some cases, for instance, the invented socially superior ways of behaving would mark some people off from their social inferiors. Such modes of behaviour might become more generally accepted in society. But such reasons merely explain why rules of etiquette exist. They do not justify these rules; they do not give us any reason to think that these rules should be accepted rather than some others. If someone pressed for a reason why fingers are held this way when drinking tea from a china cup, it would be perfectly acceptable to reply: 'That is just how things are'. There is no further reason to continue in this way. The rules of etiquette can be arbitrary.

Moral principles, in contrast, cannot be arbitrary. There will always be some explanation of how people hold their moral views. But in addition it is plausible that it is part of 'morality' that if someone thinks that people ought, morally, to behave in a certain fashion, he or she can be asked to give reasons why people should behave in this fashion. Someone who thinks, for instance, that a doctor ought (or ought not) to be wholly truthful with his or her clients — and thinks this is a moral principle — had better have some reason for this conviction. It would not be enough to reply to someone who challenged the principle: 'That is how we do things in this Health Authority'. However things are done in one hospital, or authority, or country, people in another place may think — on moral grounds — that they should be done differently.

Implicit in this is a second difference. The norms of etiquette are relative; the norms of morality are not. Belching at the dinner table is distinctly bad form; however there are societies in which it is considered perfectly acceptable — indeed it is regarded as a way of complimenting the host or hostess. This thought may be distasteful initially, but there are two differ-

ent ways of going on, each of which is perfectly acceptable. Rules of
etiquette in one society are not 'correct', any more than rules in other
societies are 'incorrect'. Belching at the dinner table is 'acceptable'
behaviour in one society and not acceptable in another. There is no question that either of these societies has got it 'right' or 'wrong'.

The rules of etiquette, therefore, are relative. They differ from society
to society, and are neither 'correct' nor 'incorrect'. Morality is not relative
in this way.

Moral norms often differ between societies as rules of etiquette. Often,
a superficial difference overlies a more profound similarity. For instance,
it is repeated in books of moral philosophy that some eskimaux think it
right to leave their old people to die in the snow, whereas some people
think this quite horrific behaviour. On reflection in some circumstances
this is morally correct behaviour for eskimaux. The moral principle that
'old people deserve the best' will require different modes of behaviour in
different circumstances. This is a general, and important, truth about
moral principles. This is not a genuine difference in moral norms. Different
societies sometimes have different moral norms, just as they have different
rules of etiquette. That is as far as the similarity goes however. If there is
a society that thinks it morally alright to, say, keep slaves, or practise
clitoridectomy because it is customary, then that is a moral difference
between one society and others. This is not the same as a difference of
etiquette. Of course, keeping slaves may be alright in that society but not
in others; but this is simply a misleading way of saying that it is considered
alright in one society but not in another. In this sense moral norms differ
from society to society. But in addition to the question of what different
moral norms exist in different societies, there is a further question: which
of these moral norms is 'correct'? Whereas etiquette is relative, morality
is universal.

Which moral norms are correct? People think of their own norms (by
which they do not necessarily mean those of their society) as correct. This
is what it is for them to be 'theirs'. Some modesty is due here however,
as elsewhere, when one's view differs from those of others. Moral norms,
unlike the norms of etiquette, are neither relative nor arbitrary.

MORALITY AND CUSTOM

Morality also contrasts with another set of norms, a wider set than that
of etiquette, namely custom. The custom in most of the Western world
nowadays is for men to wear trousers, and women to wear skirts. This
has some normative effects. Children do not have free choice in the
matter. Until recent times, there were large social pressures against women
wearing trousers. But there is no good reason why people should dress
in this way rather than in some other. If a small boy asks why men do

not wear skirts, there is no more reason to say to him than: 'things are like this'. Where a custom is in force, this provides people with a reason to adhere to it; a small boy in London who chose to wear a dress would be ridiculed, and that is a reason for not doing it. There is no reason, however, that justifies the custom itself; it is merely the custom.

Sometimes, when certain social practices are observed, it is not easy to be sure whether there is any reason to justify it. In unfamiliar cultures this is apparent but also in familiar cultures, as history makes clear. Modes have become 'reasons', or attempts to rationalize an attachment to what was merely a 'custom'. (The history of the relations between physicians and nurses in hospitals may provide examples of this). Often, it cannot be seen that this is a mistake, until later. If there is no reason to justify some social practice, then it is merely a custom; if there is some good reason for it, then it is not merely a custom. The difficulty in deciding whether there is any good reason for a social practice does not throw any doubt on that distinction.

Most people could think of contrasts with morality. It is customary not to tell lies, steal, rape or murder, but these things are not merely customary, since there are good reasons for refraining from these practices. Monogamy is also customary in most of the Western world. Is there any good reason for this way, rather than some other? This is a very difficult question to answer. But if there is not, then monogamy is not a moral requirement, but merely a custom.

A moral norm, simply to be a moral norm, should be backed by reasons, whereas customs and requirements of etiquette need not. The distinction between what is morally required, and what is merely customary, is an important one which people sometimes do not observe. But it does not go far towards giving a positive account of the nature of morality. The relations between morality and the law will be considered next.

MORALITY AND LAW

The criminal law is a normative system. It tells people what to do. There is some dispute about whether the civil law is a normative system; what follows refers to the criminal law. Unlike etiquette or custom, norms of a legal system cannot be merely arbitrary. No doubt a legislative body, such as the British Parliament, could enact legislation for no reason; this would still undoubtedly be 'the law'. But, unlike etiquette and custom, strong expectations exist that any legal restriction or requirement should be backed by reasons of a certain sort. A law that did not have such backing might be the law; but it would be bad law. A custom, however, is not a bad custom merely because there is no reason for it.

It is therefore no surprise that 'the law' is not relative in the same way as etiquette and custom. Laws differ from society, and not always in superficial ways. Most often, this represents different acceptable codes. If there is some society, however, in which there are laws for which no sensible reason can be given (such as, in the view of many people, laws in many societies which aim to regulate private and harmless sexual behaviour) then this may be bad law.

How, then, does the law differ from morality? Or do they in fact differ? The question of the relation between law and morality is very complicated, and there is no generally agreed view. There are people who think that morality and the law are different sorts of norm, with nothing in common. There are also people who think they are intimately related; morality may be seen as a sort of informal legal system, having exactly the same function as the law and lacking only formal procedures (enactment and coercion) found in the law. Alternatively morality be seen, not as an informal legal system, but rather an attempt to institutionalize, or enforce, morality.

Morality and the law, cover much of the same ground. It is, for instance, immoral to murder people, and also, in nearly every society, illegal. This is true for a very wide range of activities, and it seems unlikely to be merely coincidental. Morality and the law are not the same thing however. Many things are immoral because they cause harm to people (in the case of murder, the greatest harm possible). A legal system, ensures that society may be run in a reasonably ordered way, thus enabling all individuals to run their own lives free from interference from others. It is no surprise, then, that such activities as murder, theft and rape, are made illegal. So it is not merely a coincidence that murder is both immoral and illegal. Equally, the immorality and the illegality of murder are different. If Parliament decreed that from tomorrow murder would no long be illegal, it would, from tomorrow, no longer be illegal. It would still be immoral, however, and no decree could alter that.

There are further differences between law and morality. Morality emphasizes the inward, which the law does not. The concern of morality is with people. This is not a matter of what people do, but also of the reasons why they do it. For instance, it is of limited moral concern to morality that people frequently give to the poor; what matters is that they are motivated to do this by a concern for the plight of the poor, and not simply to enhance their own reputation. The law, however, has no concern with the inward quality of life; so long as people do not exceed the speed limit, that is all the law requires of them.

The law is relative, in a way in which morality cannot be. In the USA it is, in some states, illegal to sell mechanical means of contraception except to those who have a doctor's prescription; in most states it is not illegal. The morality of contraception is not like this however; either it is immoral, or it is not. It is not immoral in one society, and morally acceptable in another. This is not to deny that it might be thought immoral in one society, but not in another, or that circumstances might make it immoral in one society but not in another.

It is also hard to resist the conclusion that the law is subject to moral requirements. A legal system may be thought morally defective in several ways. It may, for instance, use legal processes which are unjust. Under the Nazi regime in Germany, some laws were enacted in secret; it was thus impossible to know whether a person was breaking the law or not. Actual laws may violate the rights of citizens. Laws governing private, mutually consenting, sexual behaviour do this. In both of these cases, the law itself is morally defective; morality and the law must in some sense be distinct.

Morality is a system of norms, universal application, backed by reasons. It is not unusual for people, when asked the reason why they think some mode of behaviour (abortion, for example) is immoral, to reply that they think it immoral because it is against their religion. What does this mean? Is it a good reason?

MORALITY AND RELIGION

People who state that abortion is immoral because it is against their religion may mean: 'It is immoral simply because God forbids it'. This very common response is inadequate. This is not just because religious beliefs are not universally, or even widely, shared. This has often been taken, however, to be a good reason not to try to found morality on religion. Its inadequacy was pointed out more than two thousand years ago by the Greek philosopher Plato (Tredennick, 1954). If someone holds that abortion is morally wrong because God forbids it (and generally, that whatever is morally right or wrong is so because God requires or forbids it), then the following dilemma exists: did God forbid abortion because it is morally wrong, or is abortion morally wrong, simply because God forbade it?

If the first alternative is true (which is the alternative most often accepted by Christian thinkers) then this presupposes a standard of morality independent of God. There is some reason why abortion is wrong and that God, being all-knowing, knows what this reason is and, has reliably commanded people not to do it. In this case, the reason why abortion is wrong is not simply that God forbids it. Attention shifts to the question of why abortion is wrong: what is the reason? It is hard not to think that, whatever that reason may be, it should be a reason valid for everyone, whatever their religious beliefs. After all, the religious believer will not want to think that it is alright for an atheist woman to have an abortion, simply because she is an atheist.

The second alternative states that abortion is wrong simply because God forbids it. It is not that God has any reason for forbidding abortion; it is 'arbitrarily wrong'; many people do not find this a pleasant or believable picture. It raises the question why God should forbid something that there is no logical reason to forbid; this sounds like the behaviour of a deranged tyrant, rather than a God. It also has the following consequence: if God had not forbidden abortion, then there would have been nothing wrong with it, since its wrongness is wholly a matter of God having forbidden it. Anyone who thinks that abortion is wrong is unlikely to accept this.

The first alternative generally has been more acceptable. Accepting this alternative serves a link thought to exist between morality and religion. Religions generally do contain a moral dimension, and different religions often make different moral demands. This is not surprising; religions usually have a general cultural identity of their own, and their moral dimension is a part of this. Moral beliefs do not depend upon religious beliefs however. If someone holds a moral belief that abortion is wrong then he or she should have some reason for this; and simply to say that it is against his or her religion will not count as a reason.

If some behaviour is morally 'wrong', then there must be reasons for thinking this. The reasons that people generally accept as relevant to morality can be broadly classified into two types. There are appeals to welfare, or what is in people's interests. It is usually considered relevant to the moral assessment of an action that it makes people better or worse off. Problems in medical ethics illustrate this.

CONFIDENTIALITY

The much-discussed question of confidentiality in medicine is one example. In 1971 the General Medical Council decided whether a doctor in Birmingham had been guilty of 'serious professional misconduct' (the case is discussed in Veatch, 1981). He had disclosed to the father of a teenage client that she had been prescribed an oral contraceptive by the Birmingham Brook Advisory Centre, despite the fact that he had been given this information in confidence by the Centre. He had neither sought (nor received) the person's permission to disclose it. The case was complicated, but the nub of the defence was that the doctor had acted in the girl's best interests. He said that he had had two motives in informing the parents. One was the physical hazards of the 'pill', and the second was the associated moral and psychological hazards. He was found not guilty.

The GMC had to decide whether the doctor's action was 'professional misconduct', which is not the same as immorality. Professional ethics, (the contravention of which constitutes professional misconduct) are, however, a branch of general ethics. Nursing ethics, for instance, is the branch of ethics which deals with the problems that are characteristic of the situation of nurses. In effect, the doctor had been accused of immorality. It was regarded as relevant to whether his action was 'right' or 'wrong' that it had been done in the best interests of his client. It was done to further her welfare. Whatever else might be said, most people might conclude that this was a relevant consideration.

The relationship of welfare to morality is controversial. There is an ethical theory (utilitarianism) which holds that 'welfare' is a matter of pleasure and pain. In any situation, the right action is one which produces the greatest amount of welfare for all people who are affected by it (Smart, 1961). Other ethical theories have a more expansive conception of welfare. Whatever that phrase may mean, it is not just a matter of whether clients are made happy or unhappy, or whether they get in life what they want.

WELFARE

The notion of welfare is very vague; it is a cause of serious moral problems. Most people, unlike utilitarians, think that a person's welfare is made up of several different elements that can conflict. Moreover, there is no settled agreement as to what these elements are. An example will make both points clearer.

It is in a person's interests not to die. It is also in a person's interest not to be in pain. A familiar problem in medicine is that sometimes a person may be in such a condition that it is not possible to further both interests. What should be done? It is no answer to say that the decision should be with the individual. All concerned may find themselves in a dilemma with no obvious solution. Equally, the patient concerned may know exactly which course seems preferable; this illustrates the second aspect of this vagueness. What counts as being 'in a person's interest' is something that different people will decide differently. Someone may think that life is valuable, even when the cost is immense pain; someone else may feel differently. Others may not know what to feel. In another context, some people would feel that certain sexual practices were not in an individual's (best moral) interest, even if these practices led to no sort of harm or unhappiness. Others would deny this.

It is appropriate to classify all of these concepts of welfare together by comparison of moral reasoning based on welfare with another, radically different, sort. The case of confidentiality will be a useful illustration. It may have been in the best interests of the doctor's client that her parents should know of her intention to have a sexual relationship with her boyfriend. This, however, does not simply settle the matter. There is something other than her welfare to consider; the information had been given in confidence, and people have a right that confidences should not be broken. To break someone's confidence is to violate one of their rights. This is not just because it is not in someone's interest that a confidence be broken. Quite the reverse; it is easy to imagine cases where it is in someone's interest that their confidence is broken. A conflict exists: one course of action will further someone's welfare, but violate his or her rights, whereas the other course will respect those rights, but not further the person's welfare. One problem that may face a physician is knowing whether disclosure is in the person's best interest. If it can be determined that it is in the person's best interest however then this simply produces a new, and more difficult, dilemma: should one respect the person's rights, or further their welfare?

Those people who think that morality is entirely a matter of welfare do not, of course, have to face this dilemma; in their view, so-called 'rights' have no moral weight. Equally, there have been moral theories which accord welfare no moral weight. These moral theories hold that there are certain actions which simply ought not to occur whether or not it would be in someone's interest. So, for instance, it might be held that people ought not to tell lies or break a promise, or betray a confidence, even if someone's welfare (or people's welfare in general) could be furthered by doing any of these things. Such theories may take different forms. The most influential form nowadays (and the most influential amongst writers on medical ethics) is that people have certain rights, (legitimate demands against the behaviour of other people), and that these rights ought not to be violated. Some of these rights may be rights to certain levels of welfare (such as the right to a certain standard of living) but others may have nothing to do with welfare. People have a right to run their own lives, free from the paternalistic interference of others, even when this is not in their best interests. This is often referred to as the right to autonomy. Anyone who thinks this is also likely to think that being lied to (or having confidences betrayed), even when this is in their best interest, is a violation of rights and morally wrong.

There are moral theories which give exclusive weight to the demands of welfare, and moral theories, which deny any weight at all to these demands. The moral thinking of most people is not like either. Most people will think that the demands of welfare do have moral weight, but also there are certain rights to be respected, even when 'respecting' them is not in someone's best interest. This conflict between rights and welfare is the major cause of some of the most acute moral problems in health care. The dilemma it poses can be acute; although it need not be. Sometimes the right which is violated may be particularly important, whereas the gain in welfare may be enormous. People often think, for example, that children and minors do not have a very strong right to confidentiality. Sometimes people feel that when values conflict, there are simply conflicting reasons for action, both having weight, but with no obvious way of comparing the weight of each reason. Thus there seems no way of deciding what is the 'right course of action' when such a conflict occurs.

RIGHTS

In uncertain circumstances, people should use their own judgement. Since different people weigh the demands (of welfare and rights) differently, then sometimes they will judge differently; when they do, then there is no possibility of further discussion. Exactly what is meant by 'judgement' here is not clear. If there is no way of comparing the weight of the reasons, exercising judgements is difficult. Sceptics may say that if people genuinely feel pulled in both directions, they may as well toss a coin. There can be no generally agreed formula for solving these conflicts. Each person must decide for him or herself.

Morality is principled; it operates with some general principles that apply to all cases. It is also indeterminate — the principles do not always determine clearly what is right and what is wrong. This requires the exercise of judgement.

This is the open-endedness of morality. Since the world is always changing, however complete our moral thinking may seem to be, it will not cover all possible cases. Medicine provides a striking illustration.

Advances in medicine pose new ethical problems which have not been thought about before. It will be possible, by genetic engineering, to choose the nature of children. No more fundamental moral principles than those already known are required to think about the moral problems raised by this possibility. The welfare of prospective children, their parents, the welfare of society, the rights of parents, of the prospective children, and of the professionals who will be asked to complete this genetic engineering, should be considered, as should our responsibilities to future generations. There is nothing new in these principles. How they apply to this particular problem is another matter, however, and one that has not been given serious thought since it had not so far been a serious problem. It is a new ethical problem (Glover, 1984).

New ethical problems are always possible; the world is always changing in unpredictable ways and people will be faced continually with ethical problems they have not previously thought about. Moreover, the rate of change is increasing. The past two centuries have brought advances in technology in excess of anything that occurred in the previous history of humankind. This is one reason, though not the only one, why there is now less moral consensus, and more sense of the difficulty of moral dilemmas, in the developed world. Technological advance is not likely to slow down, so the 'open-mindedness' of morality is important.

PROFESSIONAL ETHICS

Professional ethics, generally, have developed recently in both academic philosophy and in the professions. This is an expression of the need from

many professionals for guidance with ethical problems. There are complex
reasons why this need has begun to be more urgent. In the medical
profession one reason has been new ethical problems. How much
guidance with ethical problems can codes of professional ethics
provide?

They cannot provide as much as people often expect. The nature of
moral reasons illustrates this, in particular the issue of confidentiality. The
UKCC Code of Professional Conduct requires nurses to:

> Respect confidential information obtained in the course of professional
> practice and refrain from such information without the consent of the
> patient/client, or a person entitled to act on his/her behalf, except where
> disclosure is required by law or by the order of a court or is necessary
> in the public interest.

(UKCC, 1985)

In some respects, this is admirably clear. Assuming that respecting of
confidential information requires people not to divulge it, then this would
prohibit any disclosure which was motivated by a concern for the interests
of the person. Paragraph one however requires the nurse to: 'Act always
in such a way as to promote and safeguard the wellbeing and interests of
patients/clients'. This seems, in contrast, to require divulgence in such
cases. Problems arise, however, with the last six words: '**necessary in the
public interest**'. The idea is clear: the patient's (*sic*) right to confidentiality
can be overridden when it is necessary in the interest of the public. But —
unless this is to be taken absolutely literally — this does not really give
any moral guidance. There are cases where the seriousness and urgency
of a threat to the public interest would morally require overriding the
person's right to confidentiality. But how serious, and how urgent, does
the threat have to be? There is deep and widespread disagreement about
this and it is hard to envisage things differently.

Codes that rule on these disagreements would face two problems.
Firstly, it would be hard to know how to phrase the ruling. It would be
no good to say that the threat to the public interest need be serious. This
would simply raise the question: what exactly is a serious threat? This is
another moral matter, about which there is widespread disagreement.
This is not to deny there are many things that would be widely agreed a
serious threat; it is simply to say that many would not. Help could be
provided by giving specific examples and rulings on these examples. This
would be extremely cumbersome however; nurses could not spend their
time trying to familiarize themselves with a voluminous case law.

There is a second problem. Clear and definitive rulings could be made
on these issues and embodied in a code; however, many people in the
profession would find themselves in disagreement with the rulings. It is
the deep disagreement about these matters that raised the original prob-

lem. A code of ethics would not make this go away, it would merely foster disaffection in the profession. Many people would find disclosure was 'against their conscience'; they would disobey it and face the threat of disciplinary action if they did. If a ruling specifically required such disclosures, then others would find themselves in the same position. In some cases, a code acceptable to the profession simply will not be able to make any definitive ruling.

Both problems are general. So long as professional codes are required to give moral guidance then they are inescapable. What professional codes cannot give is precisely what many people would like them to give. Everyone must decide for him or herself about morality.

This is not to say that professional codes have no function. There are several things that they can do.

They might simply pledge the nurse (or other professional) to the highest standards of care, without trying to settle difficult ethical questions about appropriate ways to care for people. They would then need to be framed very generally. Such a code would not give specific moral guidance, but simply require the nurse to adopt a serious and responsible attitude to moral problems that might arise. This might serve some purpose, as 'pledges' elsewhere (in courts of law, for instance) are thought to work. It would not require nurses to decide moral problems in any particular way. It might make them take these issues more seriously. This is all the person has a right to expect.

Some people may find this unsatisfactory: They might prefer greater uniformity in the profession, both for the protection of clients (who know what they can expect), and nurses (who know precisely what is required of them). Professional codes then will need to be more like legal codes than moral codes. In particular, they will need to be long and detailed, and they will have to take a stand (as the law sometimes does) on issues that morally divide the profession. They must not give moral guidance on such issues; quite the reverse. They must sometimes abstract from the question of what is morally right and wrong and decide (on other grounds) what is considered acceptable professional behaviour.

For reasons already given there could not be any code of this sort acceptable to whole profession. Some topics will have to be left to the moral judgement of the individual professional. Most professions currently have codes which (when taken in conjunction with the commentary and case-law that disciplinary bodies produce, as they enforce their professional codes) serve both functions. Vagueness and compromise exist where the issues are morally most difficult. Given the nature of moral problems, this would seem to be inevitable.

REFERENCES

Glover, J. (1984) *What Sort of People Should There Be?* Pelican, Harmondsworth.

Smart, J. J. C. (1961) *An Outline of a System of Utilitarian Ethics*. Melbourne University Press, Melbourne. Rpt. in *Utilitarianism: For and Against* by J. J. C. Smart, Cambridge University Press.

Tredennick, H. (ed.) (1969) *Plato: The Last Days of Socrates*. Penguin, London.

UKCC (1985) *Code of Professional Conduct for the Nurse, Midwife and Health Visitor*. United Kingdom Central Council for Nursing, Midwifery and Health Visiting, London.

Veatch, R. (1981) *A Theory of Medical Ethics*. Basic Books. New York.

Chapter Three

Ideological themes in mental health nursing

LIAM CLARKE

EDITORS' INTRODUCTION

Contemporary practice does not exist in a vacuum: we are all part of history and can influence other's history. Our ideas about care, treatment and helping are, at least in part, a function of history. The ideas which shape contemporary practice were themselves once shaped by now out-moded practices. Society's need to distance itself from people with mental health problems produced the asylum tradition and, in time, the birth of modern psychiatry. Many major, early influences on 20th century psychiatry, merely translated older prejudices into theoretical standpoints: Jaspers maintained that 'no great human difference' could exist than between the normal person and the 'psychotic'. Harry Stack Sullivan later felt impelled to state his belief that 'psychotics' were, more than anything else, 'simply human'. Whatever kind of care or treatment people with mental health problems need, we should not forget to treat them, however different they may be from us, as 'simply human'.

In this chapter **Liam Clarke** considers the ideas which may have shaped psychiatric nurses' practices, and also the ideas which they own. These 'personal ideologies' may have obscure disparate sources but are, nonetheless, important influences on the practice of care. To what extent do these important members of the mental health service treat those in their care as simply human?

Ideological themes in mental health nursing

Nursing historians have dealt with general hospital nursing, (i.e. medico-surgical nursing) with barely a passing glance at the asylum or at mental nurses. A few (otherwise excellent) books purport to be histories of nursing, but virtually deny the existence of a large undergrowth of mental nursing, preferring to examine the kinds of nursing (and nurses) which the public have come to know and revere.

More effective than this 'minimization' process, however, is the manner of story-telling. Reverential writing has been greatly enhanced by a biographical approach to nursing history. A 'famous figures model' (Carpenter, 1980) is utilized to obliterate the intellectual and practical concerns of those who occupy 'the shop floor' of nursing. Mental nursing is subsumed beneath stories of the progressive reforms of this or that leader; the mental patients of Britain — or what they might represent — and their 'carers' are kept at literary arm's length. This denial is continued by the high ideals of a minority, who articulate in press, whilst not inhabiting the workplaces of the majority in any physical or psychological sense.

HISTORICAL BACKGROUND — 19TH TO 20TH CENTURY

From the 19th century, attendants lived very closely in time and place to the 'pauper lunatics' whose wretched existence they jealously maintained — perhaps as a reflection of their own occupational misery. Often perceived as little different to their charges, the attendants might yet respond towards them with indiscriminate punitiveness (Ulmann, 1967). Their attitudes and behaviours appear to have been governed by a need to construct a social system whereby they might obtain a nugget of power and control over the lunatics (Belknap, 1956), in the name of service to a revered (but hated) medical profession.

The origins of this compliance revolve around issues of social class, gender and education. In the Nightingale era, nurses were by no means uniform in terms of social class, but amongst their numbers were both middle class women and 'ladies' of good education. Abel-Smith (1960) records that these women, generally, were of higher social class than doctors working in the same hospitals. Fearing that these educated women would undermine their authority, the doctors protested, successfully, the need for a medical-prescriptive sphere of influence. Men were unwelcome as general nurses and, at the turn of the century, almost all were employed in the mental asylums. Pilgrim (1988) notes that men who undertook nursing were perceived as socially inferior to their female counterparts, and this division was amplified by the physical restraint aspects of asylum work. Doctors feared men as potential usurpers. Male mental nurses were never permitted to develop a knowledge base, but instead were required to assimilate medical assumptions as a foundation on which to base their daily duties. In addition, possession of practical skills, absorbed via an educational curriculum based upon received ideas, led to a playing-down of theoretical or ideological debate.

It follows that an important strand of nursing ideology, formed as an aspect of the developing relationship between male attendants and doctors, was the need for an obedient and compliant patient whose '. . . only hope for approval lay in obeying orders and deporting himself as an impersonal unquestioning individual' (Bockoven, 1963).

The entire life of the patient would be organized and articulated by the attendants. This intermediary role (Towell, 1975) robbed attendants of any discretionary activities, consigning them to the base occupation of gaoler. Scheff (1966) however indicated that the intermediary role conferred enormous potential power upon the attendants, that doctors had little option but to follow their advice so that the attendants more or less ran the hospitals. Sargent (1967) graphically recounts that '. . . junior medical officers could claim no real responsibility at all' as they shuffled around wards signing numerous treatment cards. Most of these treatment cards recommended doses of bromides or paraldehyde which, despite their prescriptions, were given in poisoningly high doses anyway. When not doing this they were signing detention orders on request from attendants.

The relationship of the attendants to the junior doctors significantly indicates the stifling strength of the lunatic asylum ideology. Whatever the tendencies of some junior doctors to question the 'system', they seemed overpowered by the sheer weight of numbers of both nursing staff and clients, as well as the intimate 'knowledge' which these two groups shared. There is little evidence that junior doctors tried to change things, instead deciding to leave (as Sargent did) or blindly accept their lot. The nurses dreaded change and invested huge, probably half-mythical, powers in the medical superintendent; it was he (*sic*), who would punish any misdemeanour or infringement of 'the rules'. That the superintendents possessed wide-ranging and swingeing powers is not in doubt. This was achieved without procedures of enforcement, other than long and meticulous rule-books (Carpenter, 1980).

There existed, between the attendants and superintendents, a symbiotic relationship in support of the colony-asylum and its inhabitants; and a determination, on the part of the attendants, to resist interference or change. There emerged a cringeing belief in the sublimity of sameness: a living ideology of doing things which had always been (and would always be) done. The evolution of management-disciplinary procedures, coupled with the developing strength of male-oriented trade-unionism restructured, but essentially sustained, this ideology — persons validating each others' performances — as responses to institutional requirements.

In this way questions of authority and relationships, especially elements of sexuality and aggression, continued to be defined as problems to be 'dealt with' rather than as social or psychological phenomena which needed to be understood. Both sides secretly needed each other so as to devalue forms of therapeutic inquiry or evaluation; such therapeutic activities might result in assault or injury to their common perspective (and need) for power. The construction of client/nurse interactions took shape within this insensitive field (Altschul, 1972; Ashworth, 1980) with human relationships becoming subject to the asylum regime (Goffman, 1961) and with potential conflict (or insurrection) contained, or at least confined.

FEAR AND CONTAINMENT

The central perception of the client, therefore, was that he or she was a lunatic; not so much an 'object model' (Mcfarlane, 1982) but rather a kind of inferior and primitive being who, if unleashed, would wreak havoc upon his or her unprotected fellows. Containment was a protective mechanism easily adopted by attendants, who were to play a greater role in containing 'madness' (*sic*) than any other group (Bell, 1954; Macmillan, 1956; Rees, 1956). Reserving to themselves a 'self-serving rationality' (Foucault, 1961) they subdued aggression — especially of a sexual kind — within an extraordinary array of chores and rituals.

Certainly the ever-present need for a 'well-run ward', Spartan, clean and predictable (like a good conscience) may have driven the attendants to perceive imminent conflict and dissolution as outside of themselves and in desperate need of control. Repeatedly nurses projected their worst fears on to their demoralized patients. Extending the metaphor, it may be that 'lunatic containment' symbolized some measure of the containment of social insanity; the lunatic, stripped of social meaning, became a perfect transference model. Shoenberg (1980) referred to hospitals as 'castles of fantasy' embroiling all within (and without) their walls, the central notion of these fantasies being the hospital-as-container for the 'wild threatening part of ourselves' and the ever-present danger of loss of control.

For the general public the 'terrifying and rejecting self' is projected into a safe place, locked up and always far away. For the nurses, of course, it remained close enough to smell, the projected dangers visible in the faces of those who are the principal receptors of society's madness, the clients. The management of projective fears is tenuous at best and activities, both internal and external, may be evolved — becoming more 'progressive' and socially acceptable over time — to make the environment safe. It is from such fusions of communal fear that therapies must spring, whose chief manifestation may be that of professionalized helping, but whose latent motive may be some form of control.

Since containment can serve several functions, and take different forms, as time passed, the emerging ideologies of nursing necessarily altered from hospital and public pressures. For instance, the provision of work and industrial 'therapies' often served as an inducement to stay, rather than for any intrinsic value they might possess: 'After all why should a patient leave the only place where he can always be sure of a kind word and a sympathetic ear?' (Stern, 1957).

Similarly when, 'The walls came tumbling down' (Mapperley Hospital Centenary History, 1880–1980), more tentacle-like controls took their place,

such as parole systems, and an ever-burgeoning vocabulary and parapher-
nalia of 'modern psychiatry'.

The evolution of 'attendants' into 'nurses' maintained the priority given
to the changing currencies of medical requirements. For example, nurses
rarely (if ever) question their relationship to the administration of drugs.
Rather, they continue to be given to patients simply because they are
prescribed. (The ongoing battle with junior medical personnel is seen in
the expressed annoyance at 'too low' dosages of drugs prescribed by the
juniors.) Most nurses value drug prescriptions, because they cement the
perceived necessity of a medical model pact with psychiatry. Nurses, in
this instance, have been described as 'fellow travellers' (Pilgrim, 1988),
although this seems to diminish the intrinsic element of nursing intent
involved in their collusion (Stein, 1978). Such intent was clarified in the
move from hospital to local settings where too few nurses had regard for
this, other than as a shift of resources and power. Wider therapeutic
networks might have been expected to demonstrate more potent socio-
political responses other than depot-injection clinics, and the laboured
language of simplistic psychotherapies (Clarke, 1989).

There has been a peculiar inability to achieve more than a moderate
articulation of the growing desperation of socially-deprived, discharged
hospital clients. With very few exceptions, the community psychiatric
nursing literature reveals the apolitical stance endemic to classical British
psychiatry (Community Psychiatric Nursing Journal 1984–1987; Simpson,
1989). There is even an occasional declaration of 'ideological neutrality',
such as Carr's (1984) claim that the anti-psychiatric activities of some
community psychiatric nurses was: '. . . a case of pragmatism rather than
a counter-ideology changing with established patterns of practice'.

There have been attempts, by some community nurses, to achieve a
measure of clinical autonomy but, in addition to lack of resources, these
activities also have been hampered by the transposition of traditional
administrative structures from hospital to local settings.

Nurses are quick to deny much of this nowadays, espousing a 'nursing
process' or other psycho-social model. But whilst they may indeed modu-
late their 'medical model' in variegated responses to a person's problems,
this strategy perfectly matches the 'me too' eclecticism of much modern
psychiatry. It continues to validate its position through assimilation
(Baruch and Treacher, 1978) and feigned pragmatism, whilst always holding a physical treatment in reserve. There exists a 'lip service' approach
to psycho-social nursing tortuously concealed in much of the literature on
'therapeutic nursing'. Occasionally truer, if unwitting, glimpses of the
actual state of play can be seen:

Now the role of the mental illness nurse approximates more closely to
the role of the general nurse in that the psychiatrists need nurses to

support and care for patients whilst their prescribed treatment takes
effect and to care fully for patients when their treatment is of limited or
no avail.

(Stockwell, 1985)

The reality is that nurses have associated themselves with a safe and
accessible 'biological defect ideology' of mental illness — much enhanced
by the supposed 'revolutionary' effects of the phenothiazine drugs
(Ramon, 1985). This largely precluded the possibility of recovery, and
appeared to equate the dilapidated and pathetic state of their clients as
both inevitable and unworthy of an intelligent or even humanitarian
response (Barton, 1957; John, 1961; Ulmann, 1967; Beardshaw, 1981;
Martin, 1984; Lunder, 1987).

THE REIGN OF CONFUSION

The degree of insightful obeisance to the medical profession, or other
structures, is open to question. Physicians are a group unable (or unwilling) to examine, in any form, what they are doing, preferring,
'. . . unanalysed customs . . . where tradition is adhered to rigidly . . .
and change implies threat . . .' (Barber, 1989). To assert, as many do, that
nurses base their practices on abstract philosophies is 'probably naive'
(Wilson and Kneisl, 1988): treatment ideologies are intertwined with the
everyday realities of the work situation. This was evident in the study
which identified three major orientations, namely: an analytical-psycho-
therapeutic ideology; an organic-directive ideology and a socio-therapeutic
ideology. Nurses' attitudes were dispersed throughout these ideologies
and were unable to perceive differences between them. Altschul (1972) in
turn suggested that nurses did not possess any identifiable perspective to
guide them in their dealings with problematic issues. Nurses may be
unwilling (or unable) to assert themselves therapeutically, in relation to
other disciplines.

Another description of the effects of 'ward ideology' (whether custodial,
medical or therapeutic community) with respect to how nurses conducted
themselves, suggested that they appeared to suffer greatest difficulty in
the 'therapeutic community', where they would be least subject to task
or role 'direction', whilst under some obligation to make an individual
contribution (Towell, 1975). An earlier study had commented on the presence of 'psychological distance' in therapeutic communities, which was
due to incomplete acceptance of therapeutic community ideology by the
nurses (Caine and Smail, 1968). This tendency to 'get on with the job' and
to be seen to do so — the belief that there was a discrete job or task to
be done — militated against 'trivial' interactions with people who were
perceived as mad, and therefore beyond ordinary social intercourse.

The relative absence of discussion and reflection, as opposed to 'doing' (including ward office-based writing), has occasionally been recognized as a general phenomenon. Caudill *et al.* (1952) has shown that nurses 'spoke less'. Davis (1981) demonstrated an 'inadequacy in conversation' amongst nurses, as well as a reluctance to enter lengthy conversations. More recently, White (1985) stated that theoretical or ideological discussion had not been a major preoccupation amongst psychiatric nurses. A more profound level of nurses' silence, however, may be that of unwillingness to change; an 'inarticulate speech of the heart', born of resentment to change, and its concomitant anxieties (Clark, Hooper and Oram, 1962).

These unspecified (but widespread) fears and practices were rarely included in a growing 'research' activity which, with great determination, described psychiatric nursing from the vantage point of *a priori* concepts and theories, with little attention to ward-based realities, 'harsh' or otherwise. 'Thus, the prescriptive and descriptive literature relating to the role of the psychiatric nurse do not coincide, nurses do not appear to be doing what the literature suggests they ought to be doing' (Cormack, 1983).

The attention to discrepancies between 'reality' and research literature has added to the confusion. Prescriptive writing is rarely defined as such, and may masquerade as reality-based. Altschul (1985), for example, asserted that: 'since a medical model leads predominantly to the use of drugs this aspect of care will not be discussed.' She asserted that British nurses have been concerned with models based on psychological and social theories. The truth, however, probably lies closer to where patients are 'housed', and with those whose responsibility it is to house them:

> The professional requirements of nurses appear to lose out more often since the nurses had to get the work done, do business as usual, and push medications in the name of treatment in order to facilitate easy discharge to free a number of limited beds for incoming patients.
>
> (Haugen-Bunch, 1985)

THE OFFICIAL ENQUIRY AS RESEARCH

Nursing histories have continued publicly to enshrine highly circumscribed definitions of nursing, until at least the 1980s (Carpenter, 1980). Some truths had begun to seep out, however horribly and grudgingly, in the mid–1960s via the activities of concerned individuals and groups. These included that time-worn stimulus to change, letters to the press (Jones, 1972), investigative journalism, and the assertions of individuals from within British mental hospitals. These people were called 'insiders' (Martin, 1984) to distinguish them from the 'outsider' (non-professional) authors of a more disturbing and disturbed book (Robb, 1967). This book was discredited, with relative ease, by showing its technical inaccuracies, and by urbanely dismissing its emotional heart-cries as malicious and/or seditious.

Allegations made by small numbers of nurses, both to nurse-managers (and subsequently to the press) were not, however, so easily blanketed. These 'insiders' were, 'outsiders' by virtue of their relative lack of institutionalization, or indoctrination, so that they persisted in their criticisms and would not stop; they tended to occupy the lower regions of pathetically proud and stultifying nursing hierarchies; often they were nursing assistants, students, or part-time working women whose views, by definition, would be regarded as those of the ignorant, the inexperienced or immature (Martin, 1984). As 'whistle-blowers' (Beardshaw, 1981) they left themselves vulnerable to varying degrees of personal abuse and hierarchical vilification. They would have been unaware that high-ranking nurses at the DHSS were fully aware (and had been for some years) of the abuses which could (and did) exist within their highly secretive hospitals (Martin, 1984). With little hope of support, and with much derision, they publicized a shocking agenda of cruelty, neglect, and therapeutic perversion which, whatever the ideological constraints of institutional existence, was only believable as a result of years of social, historical and 'professional' cover-up, ably contained within the furtive comradeship of male-dominated trade unions and their time-worn alliance with 'management'.

A long series of public inquiries into mental hospital services has occurred, although careful reading of these reports reveals a minority of blatant wrongdoers (see Miller and Gwynne, 1972). An uneasy feeling exists that it would have been impossible for everybody not to have known what was going on: the stunning callousness and heartlessness of (predominantly male) nurses treating their 'victims' as if they were a lower form of animal life. That these outrages obtained general acquiescence may also be explained by the ferocious responses directed towards the few people ('lower down' the nursing hierarchy) who did not acquiesce. Even physical attack occurred (Martin, 1984) and public/professional disgrace anticipated by those at the top if found out.

The absence of 'proper' research leaves matters inconclusive (for some); Jones (1972) for example, implicitly exonerated all hospitals in her discussion. In an extraordinary appeal directed at those who occupy 'high moral ground' Taylor (1983) referred to the: '. . . rare violence of a nurse [as] an unavoidable vocational hazard . . .' and offered a mixture of difficult clients and indifferent managers as an acceptable justification for brutality.

It is not possible to deny many of the intolerable conditions which Taylor (1983) described; nevertheless there exists a universal foundation of knowledge which takes account of far more than provoked 'unfortunate' violent incidents. The examination of the nature and form of some of the abuses suggests it occurred in many mental hospitals.

HIERARCHIES

A predominant feature of nursing hierarchies has been their inherent powers of sanction. Students, as well as qualified staff, have traditionally regarded the hospital wards (and not the nursing school) as 'the real world' and have, usually, invested its more elaborate hierarchy with potentially greater powers of sanction. But although liberal sentiments may be expressed within the sterile contexts of teaching situations, it is rare for students to personify any ideological or ethical problems by a process of naming names.

Beardshaw (1981) looked at outcomes of nurses' complaints and concluded that they had good reason for keeping quiet. Junior nurses who complained were likely to be called 'troublemakers' by seniors, rather than have their complaints investigated. Few would (publicly) disagree that this is a time when students have been encouraged to develop critical acuity and awareness; a time when nurses are asked by the UKCC to become client's advocates to help to determine the most suitable treatment for them. When Les Parsons and Dee Kraaij, both student nurses, 'displayed an informed concern' (Bailey, 1983) about the use of ECT they were, however, sacked. Whilst change may be in the air, it may still prove to be dangerous. Barton (1976) talks of the covert use of punishment within nursing systems and of the dangers of being labelled 'awkward' or 'paranoid'. Tatum (1989) confirmed the overall picture of 'words unspoken' about ethical dilemmas, and the ongoing fear of the consequences of 'speaking out'. That sanctions may be less outrageous than before, does not indicate their absence.

POWER

To become a specialist in nursing is to acquire the language (and other behaviours) of a sphere of influence which is relatively distant from traditional managerial hierarchies. White (1985) has described how specialization removes the nurse from the broad base of generalist nurses who remain relatively uncritical of nursing managers. The managers, in turn, have moved to a position of control acquiring a range of generalist experiences. In the language of ordinary management, budgetary control, cost-effectiveness, performance indicators and quality assurance, they are especially mistrustful of specialists whom they have sought to suppress (White, 1985) mainly through financial control and influence of educational processes. Their objectives may owe less to any nursing ideology than to a need to achieve outcomes whose chief determinant is government dictum. To be effective, they require directive power and control. This inevitably leads them, however, towards activities which owe little to their role as a nurse. Yet if nurses are to serve clients in a manner of their choice then they need to ensure that some achieve high managerial status and power over resources.

Benner (1984) has stated that power resides in the 'power of caring' and 'excellence in caring', and that relinquishment of these nurturing activities will impede all moves towards self-determination. She has identified nurturing functions as uniquely female, and warns against aping male concepts of power, such as control and domination. Quoting from Greer (1973) she imbues women with compassion, empathy, innocence, and sensuality. Two issues have emerged; firstly, the manner in which nurses possess and exercise power and, secondly, the separation of male and female qualities.

Benner's (1984) division is an idealization of 'female' qualities in that it splits off the male role into 'executive' and 'controlling' actions. Her vision of power, through caring, is clinically confined: who defines excellence, and in relation to what yardstick? There is little need for nurses to take control of the contexts of care-delivery. Janeway (1977) has noted how 'traditional' qualities of female-hood can lead to woman-power but speaks of this as a private (individual) power for which public (collective) submission must take place. The sense of women's power, in this instance, has developed from the mythical notion of the 'giver'; although, as Janeway observes: '. . . how can one give if one does not possess riches and substance?'

Benner's (1984) idealization may be an attempt to make unbearable situations bearable, and she has added to the publicity of a 'high ideal' and 'angelic profession'. But whilst all of this may help in the acquisition of power, the exercise of power means influencing and controlling social situations where: '. . . nurses must work under conditions that are strongly influenced by economics, legislation, multiple levels of bureaucracy and paperwork . . . increased reliance on psychotropic medication, hasty discharges . . . a revolving door . . . and short stays in hospital' (Wilson, 1982).

The move away from the bed to higher management has led to an enhancement of power, to a wider social control: the dilemma resides in the loss or abrogation of the nurturing functions of nursing — assumed to be intrinsically female (Benner, 1984) — which is widely believed to go hand-in-hand with the acquisition of higher management functions (Caudhill *et al.*, 1952; Cormack, 1976).

This dilemma may operate at a variety of levels: nurses (formerly known as sisters or charge-nurses) have been redesignated ward managers and have set out to organize, evaluate and justify, often quantitatively, the delivery of nursing care. The care may be completed by those people who aspire to 'nothing more' than basic nursing care, (i.e. an ideology of vocation). The managers may aspire to an ideology of profession but, as Williams (1978) argued, this may mean the abandonment of fundamental nursing care. The suggestion is that those who nurture 'at the bedside' (in close, physical or psycho-social proximity to clients) are nurses. However, to assume that nurturing is something which goes on between two people may be misleading: one may nurture an ideal which brings fulfilment to many. The belief that nurses who achieve a 'high' status will necessarily fail to nurture ideals may be a mistake. The dilemma occurs when the art of caring for others, at whatever level, is polluted by economic and ideological constraints from a bureaucracy whose manifest agenda seems at odds with its (partially expressed) motivation. Despite the asserted benevolence of the agenda, the motivation could be identified, from a particular political viewpoint, as 'slide-rule thinking' and the ethics of the market place. Some caution is required, however; the essence of bureaucracy is that for those who function outside of it, nothing can be certain.

A UNIFIED NURSING PROFESSION

Mental nurses have never been happy with a 'common foundation preliminary training' which has followed a pattern of preparation which was too close to general nursing. In 1957 a new syllabus was formed, based on concepts of the mental hospital as a therapeutic community and an educational principle that learning had more meaning if related to particular problems faced by particular groups of nurses (Bendall and Raybould, 1969). There was a generally accepted view that certain men and women were especially suited to this work (Bendall and Raybould, 1969). British nursing developed a commitment to a psycho-social approach to training (ENB, 1982) in response to these perceived deficiencies in applying 'medical model ideologies' to mental nursing. Also, the 1982 syllabus represented a move further away from the traditional unitary concept of nursing. The implementation of the 1982 syllabus has meant that some training schools have radically altered their curricula, so that much of what remained of a medical foundation (such as drugs, diagnoses, classifications, the validity of professionalism) was dropped.

Training schools had also attracted fewer candidates for several reasons. The over-riding process of psychiatric student preparation has been based on the 'small group' of eight to ten students. These students have chosen psychiatric nursing. These circumstances suggest an educational preparation, whose common ground is with counselling and psychotherapy. This might shift radically if intake numbers increased dramatically, as is likely with the introduction of a common-foundation 'Project 2000' scheme. The resulting confusion of purpose and rationale would not be new, and it would require extensive management until the next reorganization or change.

A unified nursing profession promotes managerialism (White, 1985) and this has contributed to the defeat of grass-roots creativity and democratic change. If progressive experiments in patient care are to be integrated into a state system of care, then it is imperative that 'psychiatric tensions' be resolved in favour of non-medical psychiatric practitioners working in interdisciplinary teams. In reality, however, such teams can be oppressive and restrictive. Under the guise of libertarianism, these structures can crush innovation; truly progressive systems could function without psychiatric practitioners. Professionalization concerns are a distraction which work against the interdisciplinary goals, giving rise to problems of industrial democracy which have characterized the provision of care within the NHS (Goldie, 1977; Pilgrim, 1983). With the advent of Project 2000, yet again the concerns of many psychiatric nurses will suffer diffusion and erosion. Institutes of nursing, housing large numbers of students, teachers and curriculum planners, cannot be said to have evolved from a general consensus as to their necessity; from a therapeutic standpoint their existence remains vague. Menzies Lyth (1988) continues to talk of the 'imposition of blueprints' as further avoidance of the need to develop models from within (and as an outcome of) group processes. The current stratification of nurse education reduces the scope for decision making other than at 'the top'. The clinical-grading of nurses promotes role relationships within clearly defined hierarchical systems which also contributes to contemporary drives for professionalization and managerial 'accountability'. Nurses who are concerned with the advocacy of specific therapeutic needs, or socio-political rights, may become more marginal and drift (philosophically) ever further from current organizational trends, perhaps ultimately seceding from the mainstream altogether. The founding of such organizations as the Psychiatric Nurses Association and the Community Psychiatric Nurses Association tentatively suggests that this may already be happening.

Much of the Project 2000 discussion starts from a premise that common elements unite all nurses as a profession. Whereas there are fundamental values which most nurses share, these are pertinent to humanity as a whole; when such values are 'reduced' to attitudes which may help govern the delivery of therapy, differences may emerge and these may be measured. The head-long rush (Willmott, 1989) to implement common foundation schemes may involve a denial of significant data which suggests character and attitudinal differences existing between general and psychiatric nurses. Significant data indicating such differences (Caine, 1964; Caine and Smail, 1968, 1969; Tutt, 1970; Caine and Leigh, 1972; Abbati, 1974) is ignored by an insular nursing literature, in the drive towards a quasi-academic unified profession.

The complexity of nursing

Because nursing is so complex it is extremely difficult to find words to
make adequate sense of it.

(Stockwell, 1985, p. 11)

If you substitute the word 'complex' by 'different', you may see how easily
Stockwell gives the game away. There may be very little complexity when
nursing is viewed within specialist activities, albeit what is seen may seem
odd in the light of what is traditionally regarded as nursing. Complexity
is a euphemism for unity with its consequent imprecision and lack of
therapeutic orientation. Clarity of intent is disliked, because it obviates
the need for externally imposed frameworks; it certainly does not require
the motivation of the candidates through a network of common foundation
activities in the expectation that they will choose their specialization at
'the end'. The truth is that common foundation students will bite their
lips as they reluctantly engage in those aspects of their journey which they
perceive as irrelevant; nurses are used to deferred gratification anyway.

A caring profession

The overriding ideology of nursing has been exemplified by unremitting
appraisals of nursing as a 'generalized social activity'; a 'caring profession'
united by a common ground beloved of article-writers and high profile
spokespersons. If there is a common ground of caring, empathy, nurturing, these are also qualities possessed by some social workers, teachers,
probation officers, as well as general nurses. This could mean that there
is no such 'thing' as nursing, no uniqueness in the mix but, instead, a
mix of different therapeutic activities, often directed towards qualitatively
different ends.

The much-valued 'nursing process' assumes a generalized conceptual
status, yet has required nurses to accept a pre-determined and systematic
scheme of note-taking as effective in its denial of ambiguity as the doing
of a drug round. Nursing models are often 'need to ensure' models,
inveigling nurses into 'therapeutic' activities which often yield little more
than written accounts of 'managed' relationships to produce a 'reality' as
perfectly matched to the model as possible; students may complain when
their client fails to meet the requirements of the model.

One alternative is to stretch or adapt the model to a degree of compre-
hensiveness which renders it meaningless. Since nursing models possess
no theoretical basis, such activities are common; where the model has a
theory then it is usually borrowed. In nursing, the commonest form of
this is behaviourism. Yet if the work of a nurse who practices behaviour
therapy is indistinguishable from a psychologist who does the same, then
in what way is this nurse still a nurse? Where is the locus of unity to be

found for those psychiatric nurses, whether practitioners of behaviourism, dynamic therapy or therapeutic community? Where is the universality?

Moves towards a 'common ground' Project 2000 should be seen against the more holistic background of general nursing. Contradictions are present, however, and long-term proposals do not adequately cover those people who hold conceptions of abnormal or unusual behaviours as anything other than illness. Concepts of deviancy will be discussed, but such discussions will not lead to change, given the medically-controlled contexts of the organization, and delivery of care. This is especially true, given the sheer range of skills required of students under the planned changes. Martin (1984) has noted the fine principles of the 1982 syllabus, but it is so lengthy that nursing schools cannot cover many of the elements in depth, having to choose which subjects to emphasize.

In relation to ethnics, some schools have emphasized the person's rights, the need for individuality, and clarity about what activities of 'cruelty' are to be reported. Elsewhere the emphasis may be on traditional matters, such as correctness of dress, how to address doctors, and deference to authority. It is difficult in some of these situations to grant autonomy to clients when it is lacking in nurses; the whole picture represents much confusion. Nurses may welcome a discussion of illness as deviance or social protest, but as a kind of marginal concept: at present, if nurses choose to act upon that concept such as to implement programmes derived from it, then this too becomes a marginal activity.

The profession

In attempting to deal with such conceptual issues complications have been ignored; especially the ideological conviction of nursing as a profession, and the need to be seen in the proud companionship of other prestigious disciplines. Thus the need for unity, and a so-called body of knowledge. Few have taken heed of Salvage's (1985) ironic warning of the dangers of professions limiting knowledge to their own group. This was written at a time when 'the profession' firmly espoused the need for client-centred assessment, expression (and definition) of personal needs and mutual evaluation. On the nurse's part, empathy and genuineness require de-professionalization (Rogers, 1965). More specifically, the entire framework of 'therapeutic community nursing' is based upon the potential democracy of giving knowledge away, and living at a vaguely-defined boundary with clients. Whilst some behaviour therapists might see their knowledge in more self-possessive terms, the inference here is that if psychiatric nurses possess intra-disciplinary tensions (i.e. how to define what they are doing) then the idea of a common knowledge base which unites 'the profession' is not credible.

Those people who insist upon a 'nursing profession' have explicitly disregarded the relationship of psychiatric nurses to 'mental illness' as questions which rest on assumptions or value judgements, preferring to see mental nursing as a 'branch of the profession'. The unitary concept of nursing is aided and abetted by generalists, who make a pretence of ideological neutrality, blessed by the convention of psychiatry, whose parentage is medicine, and this permits psychiatric nursing to continue its historical role of assisting psychiatry in the medicalization of social life. This proceeds under the guise of 'demands on the profession', and the hint that, given time, scientific validation will emerge. The hidden assumptions of these views may be outlined as follows (Caine and Smail, 1969).

1. Mental health is 'objective' in that it is more than an expression of the values of the psychiatrists, or of the cultural norms of a society. It is held that mental illness is no less objective to, and analogous to, physical illness.
2. This hypothetically diagnosable mental illness may account for some socially unacceptable behaviour so that:
3. It may then diminish moral or social responsibility.

CONCLUSIONS

As Wooton (1959) pointed out, the main difficulty lies within the conflict between mental health and morals. Shotter (1975) has attempted a definition of psychological behaviour as a 'moral science of action'. Halmos (1965) has referred to the current (i.e. empathic) stance of psychotherapists to argue that this also is essentially a moral stance. Value judgements are inevitable in nursing, but they may impinge upon the work of some mental nurses in a manner which is at odds with general (or generalist) nurses. All nurses must take responsibility for their therapeutic actions, but this can only be made more visible if they attempt to define their work without too strict adherence to the problems of professionalism in society. The problems of nursing are not the result of deficiencies within individuals (Heyman and Shaw, 1984) but, rather, are due to conflicts and contradictions within the social structure of nursing which is, as it always has been, largely determined by outside forces.

REFERENCES

Abbati, V. (1974) *An Examination of Factors Related to the Selection, Success and Therapeutic Orientation of Psychiatric Student Nurses as Compared with General Student Nurses.* Unpublished Clinical Psychology Dissertation, British Psychological Society.
Abel-Smith, B. (1960) *A History of the Nursing Profession.* Heinemann, London.
Altschul, A. (1972) *Patient-Nurse Interaction.* Churchill Livingstone, Edinburgh.
Altschul, A. (1985) Annotated bibliography. In Altschul, A. (ed.) *Psychiatric Nursing.* Churchill Livingstone, Edinburgh.
Ashworth, P. (1980) *Care to Communicate.* Royal College of Nursing, London.

Bailey, J. (1983) ECT or not ECT: that is the question. *Nursing Times.* **79** (9), March 2nd, 12–14.

Barber, P. (1989) Developing the 'person' of the professional carer. Hinchliff, S. M., Norman, S. E. and Schober, J. E. (eds.) *Nursing Practice and Health Care.* Edward Arnold, London.

Barton, R. (1957) *Institutional Neurosis.* John Wright, Bristol.

Barton, R. (1976) *Institutional Neurosis,* 3rd ed. John Wright, Bristol.

Baruch, G. and Treacher, A. (1978) *Psychiatry Observed.* Routledge and Kegan Paul, Henley.

Beardshaw, V. (1981) *Conscientious Objectors At Work.* Social Audit, London.

Belknap, I. (1956) *Human Problems of a State Mental Hospital.* McGraw-Hill, New York.

Bell, G. M. (1954) The unlocked door. *Lancet,* **2**, 953–954.

Bendall, E. R. D. and Raybould, E. (1969) *A History of the General Nursing Council for England and Wales 1919–1969.* H. K. Lewis, London.

Benner, P. (1984) *From Novice to Expert.* Addison-Wesley, New York.

Bockoven, J. S. (1963) *Moral Treatment in American Society.* Springer, New York.

Caine, T. M. (1964) Personality tests for nurses. *Nursing Times.* July 24th, 973–974.

Caine, T. M. and Leigh, R. (1972) Conservatism in relation to psychiatric treatment. *British Journal of Social and Clinical Psychology,* **11**, 52–56.

Caine, T. M. and Smail, D. (1968) Attitude of psychiatric nurses to their role in treatment. *British Journal of Medical Psychology,* **41**, 193–197.

Caine, T. M. and Smail, D. (1969) *The Treatment of Mental Illness: Science. Faith and the Therapeutic Community.* University of London Press, London.

Carpenter, M. (1980) Asylum nursing before 1914: a chapter in the history of labour. In Davies, P. (ed.) *Rewriting Nursing History.* Croom Helm, London.

Carr, P. (1984) Legal and ethical perspectives in the nursing care of the mentally ill. *Community Psychiatric Nursing Journal,* **4** (5), 14–18.

Caudill, W. *et al.* (1952) Social structure and interaction process in a psychiatric ward. *American Journal of Orthopsychiatry,* **22**, (2), 314–334.

Clark, D. H., Hooper, D. F. and Oram, E. G. (1962) Creating a therapeutic community in a psychiatric ward. *Human Relations,* **15** (2), 123–147.

Clarke, L. (1989) Invention and certainty in counselling literature. *Senior Nurse,* **9** (4), 32–5; **9** (5), 32–5.

Community Psychiatric Nursing Journal, 1984–1987.

Cormack, D. (1976) *Psychiatric Nursing Observed.* Royal College of Nursing, London.

Cormack, D. (1983) *Psychiatric Nursing Described.* Churchill Livingstone, Edinburgh.

Davis, B. D. (1981) Social skills in nursing. In Argyle, M. (ed.) *Social Skills and Health.* Methuen, London.

DHSS (1969) *Report of Committee of Inquiry into Allegations of Ill-Treatment of Patients and other irregularities at the Ely Hospital, Cardiff.* HMSO, Cmnd. 3795, London.

DHSS (1971) *Report of the Farleigh Hospital Committee of Inquiry.* HMSO, Cmnd. 4557, London.

DHSS (1972) *Report of the Committee of Inquiry into Whittingham Hospital.* HMSO, Cmnd. 4861, London.

DHSS (1974) *Report of the Committee of Inquiry into South Ockendon Hospital.* HMSO, London.

ENB Syllabus: Professional Register, Part 3. (1982) English and Welsh National Board for Nursing, Midwifery and Health Visiting, London.

Foucault, M. (1961) *Madness and Civilisation: A history of insanity in the Age of Reason.* Tavistock Publications, London.

Goffman, E. (1961) *Asylums.* Penguin, Harmondsworth.

Goldie, N. (1977) The division of labour amongst the mental health professions — a negotiated or an imposed order? In Stacey, M. and Reid, M. (eds.) *Health and the Division of Labour*. Croom Helm, London.

Greer, G. (1973) Woman power. In Ogilvy, J. A. (ed.) *Self and World: Readings in Philosophy*. Harcourt Brace Jovanovich, New York.

Hall, J. N. (1974) Nurses' attitudes and specialised treatment settings: an exploratory study. *British Journal of Social and Clinical Psychology*, **13**, 333–4.

Halmos, P. (1965) *The Faith of the Counsellors*. Constable, London.

Haugen-Bunch, E. (1985) Therapeutic communication: is it possible for psychiatric nurses to engage in this on an acute psychiatric ward? In Altschul, A. (ed.) *Psychiatric Nursing*. Churchill Livingstone, Edinburgh.

Hayman, B. and Shaw, M. (1984) *Looking at relationships in nursing*. John Wiley and Sons Ltd.

Janeway, E. (1977) *Man's World, Woman's Place*. Penguin, Harmondsworth.

John, A. (1961) *A study of the Psychiatric Nurse*. Livingstone, Edinburgh.

Jones, K. (1972) *A History of the Mental Health Services*. Routledge and Kegan Paul, London.

Lunder, R. (1987) Looking back in anger. *Nursing Times*, **83** (15), 49–50.

Macmillan, D. (1956) Open doors in mental hospitals. *International Journal of Social Psychiatry*. **2** (Autumn), 152–4.

Mapperley Hospital Centenary History 1880–1980. Mapperley Hospital, Nottingham.

Martin, J. (1984) *Hospitals in Trouble*. Basil Blackwell, Oxford.

Mcfarlane, J. (1982) Nursing values and nursing action. *Nursing Times*, Occasional Paper, **78** (28).

Menzies Lyth, I (1988) *Containing Anxiety in Institutions*. Free Association Books, London.

Miller, E. J. and Gwynne, G. V. (1972) *A Life Apart*. Tavistock Publications, London.

Pilgrim, D. (1983) Politics psychology and psychiatry. In Pilgrim, D. (ed.) *Psychology and Psychotherapy: Current Trends and Issues*. Routledge and Kegan Paul, Henley.

Ramon, S. (1985) *Psychiatry in Britain*. Croom Helm, Beckenham.

Rees, T. P. (1956) Open doors in mental hospitals. *International Journal of Social Psychiatry*, **2** (Autumn), 152–4.

Robb, E. (1967) *Sans Everything: A Case to Answer*. Thomas Nelson, London.

Rogers, C. (1965) *Client Centred Therapy*. Constable, London.

Salvage, J. (1985) *The Politics of Nursing*. Heinemann, London.

Sargent, W. (1967) *The Unquiet Mind*. Heinemann, London.

Scheff, T. (1966) *Being Mentally Ill*. Weidenfield and Nicolson, London.

Shoenberg, E. (1980) Therapeutic communities: the ideal, the real and the possible. In Jansen, E. (ed.) *The Therapeutic Community*. Croom Helm, London.

Shotter, J. (1975) *Images of Man in Psychological Research*. Methuen, London.

Simpson, K. (1989) Community psychiatry nursing — a research based profession? *Journal of Advanced Nursing*, 14, 274–280.

Stein, L. (1978) The doctor-nurse game. In Dingwall, R. and Mcintosh, J. (eds.) *Readings in the Sociology of Nursing*, Churchill Livingstone, Edinburgh.

Stern, E. S. (1957) Operation sesame. *Lancet*, **1** (March 16th), 577–578.

Stockwell, F. (1985) *The Nursing Process in Psychiatric Nursing Care*. Croom Helm, Beckenham.

Strauss, A. *et al.* (1964) *Psychiatric Ideologies and Institutions*. Free Press, Glencoe.

Tatum, A. (1989) Blowing the whistle. *Nursing Times*, **85** (23), June 7th, 20.

Taylor, J. B. (1983) The tip of the lash. *Nursing Times*, **79** (42), October 19th, 72.

Towell, D. (1975) *Understanding Psychiatric Nursing*. Royal College of Nursing, London.

Tutt, N. S. (1970) Psychiatric nurses' attitudes to treatment in a psychiatric hospital. *Nursing Times*, Occasional paper, **66**, September 17th.

Ulmann, C. P. (1967) *Institution and Outcome*. Pergamon, Oxford.

White, R. (1985) Political regulators in British Nursing. In White, R. (ed.) *Political Issues in Nursing*, Volume 1. John Wiley, Chichester.

Williams, K. (1978) Ideologies of nursing: their meanings and implications. In Dingwall, R. and McIntosh, J. (eds.) *Readings in the Sociology of Nursing*. Churchill Livingstone, Edinburgh.

Willmott, Y. (1989) Letter. *Nursing Times*, **85** (23), 14.

Wilson, H. S. (1982) *Deinstitutionalised Residential Care for the Mentally Disordered: The Soteria House Approach*. Grune and Stratton, New York.

Wilson, H. S. and Kneisl, C. R. (1988) *Psychiatric Nursing*, 3rd ed. Addison-Wesley, New York.

Wooton, B. (1959) *Social Science and Social Pathology*. Allen and Unwin, London.

Part Two

Chapter Four

Psychiatry: on its best behaviour

IAN STEWART

EDITORS' INTRODUCTION

Psychiatry is a medical speciality: first defined by medical practitioners and often associated, in the eyes of the layperson, with medical doctors. The importance of psychiatrists, in the delivery of psychiatric services, should never be underestimated, but can be overstated. For the last 30 years psychiatric medicine has been called into question, however, by a significant number of dissident medical voices. 'Anti-psychiatry' is an expression of the belief that much psychiatric practice is repressive and anti-psychiatric, in the sense of a science and art concerned with 'mental healing'. The legacy of the 1960s remains, especially in the work of Italian mental health workers, mainly psychiatrists and nurses, who have tried to return the human power to people who have been dispossessed, by society and the machinery of psychiatric treatment. People with mental health problems need care and treatment: even the so-called anti-psychiatrists acknowledged this fact. But what sort of treatment?

In this chapter **Ian Stewart** reflects on the science and art of psychiatry, drawing on a long career as a psychiatrist, working in a wide range of settings. He presents an open appraisal of his experiences which clarify many of the dilemmas inherent in the doctor-patient relationship, in all its forms.

Psychiatry: on its best behaviour

An attempt at soliciting the causes of misdirection in psychiatry is seen as a logical precursor to constructive change in ethical concepts. The definition of ethics appropriate to psychiatry is the study of the specific moral choices to be made by the individual in his or her relationship with others.

Since 1970 there has been an escalation in psychiatry in agonizing over the ethical implications of the speciality. The complexities and the dilemmas inherent in this process have proved salutory, provocative and enlightening but have, predictably, produced attitudes of entrenchment, tending to negate helpful debate. Currently, the medical profession is being forced by public awareness, rather than of its own volition, to question its vulnerable moral philosophy. At the same time, psychiatry must question the constraints and distortion imposed upon its practice by the conventional alliance of medicine and psychiatry. The fundamental question is: 'Can psychiatry develop an appropriate ethical awareness within the confines of orthodox medicine?'

Many writers (e.g. Goffman, 1961; Laing, 1967; Szasz, 1974) wrongly labelled 'anti-psychiatrists' because they espouse enlightenment and change, have commented on the fragility of the ethical code in psychiatry, and express fluently and coherently their concern at the damaging ideologies within the profession. Within mental health services, ethical considerations are complicated and sometimes confused because they must be taken within the wider context of cultural changes, therapeutic reappraisals, the demands of groups over individuals, and the need to incorporate the wisdom of disparate disciplines.

In order to avoid the intellectual diversions inherent in a preoccupation with these rather academic concepts, reference is made to a statement submitted by a senior nursing administrator which encapsulates the attempted theme of this chapter.

> In my earlier days in psychiatric nursing I was at times perturbed at the lack of compassion for patients shown by certain members of the nursing staff. This resulted in a personal dilemma. I knew that incidents of this kind should be reported, but to do this would mean to stand alone against the 'closed ranks' of my colleagues. I was not at all sure how the nursing administration would react, the experience of others having shown that silence was often the best policy. I was faced with difficulties to do with witnesses of the incidents, loyalties to colleagues, future career prospects and even personal safety. I had seen things happen in the past and had no illusions about what might be done to the 'nonconformist'.

It would appear that the trouble in such a situation is that one tends not to respond immediately to one's sense that wrong is being done. Thus, the dictates of conscience become less clear and are eventually stifled to the extent that self-interest takes precedence over patient interest. 'In theory the patient comes first, but in practice this is not necessarily so' (Campbell, 1975). How could psychiatry place one of the sensitive and valuable members of its team in a situation where the best aspirations of that member had little hope of realization, save at the expense of his career, possibly his personality and, by intimation, his person?

Whether it be appreciated or appropriate, the reality of life within the mental health services is of the consultant psychiatrist holding the dominant position of power and influence. The suitability of the psychiatrist as a competent assessor of ethical problems (and this assessment) cannot be divorced from his or her clinical potential.

TRAINING

The reasons for choosing medicine as a career have been extensively researched with conclusions which correlate poorly with altruistic motivation. Nebulous unease and personal discomfort as a medical student may progress to a disturbing preoccupation when training in psychiatry. The medical curriculum does not provide adequate equipment for actually listening to people; their fears, their hopes, their goals and their true experiences are in danger of being low priority. Training may insidiously, but irrevocably, divorce people from their humanity. Psychiatrists may be taught to hear, but not to listen; to record, but not to understand; to diagnose and treat, but above all, not to feel. This training away from feeling may have a purpose; namely, an attempt to avoid being side tracked into too much awareness of others, and the implication that the sharing of the emotions of clients is an obstruction in the path to professional advancement. Therefore, in order to have true contact with clients, it may be necessary to 'untrain' and to explore areas not conventionally allied to medicine. In years of psychiatric training (which concerns itself with the so-called 'normal or well-adjusted personality') there are no discussions on which to base an opinion as to maladjustment.

Ethics as applied to mental health do not imply imposing 'happiness' on clients. The clinical objective should be to assist in the avoidance of those dilemmas which people create for themselves, through an inability to observe themselves with any degree of clarity. A preliminary to productive intervention in these circumstances should be an attempt by psychiatrists to observe themselves with clarity.

A sense of alienation within the speciality has led many psychiatrists to search both for meaning and escape. The rather apprehensive excursions into the world of semantics, theology and in particular psychology, emerged as closely allied to a purposeful, (albeit fluctuating) philosophy, which gave acceptable logic to psychiatry. On this basis of an embryonic enlightenment, an element of hope emerged in finding real communication with clients. A growing assurance developed that any interventions were less damaging, as well as an ethical awareness. In short ethical aspirations in the mental health field rested, not on learned stereotyped communication skills, but rather on communication with the client as a complete person.

A process exists by which the schoolchild hatches into the physician or psychiatrist. Restrictions imposed by science may occur at the expense of the art which derives from the individual creative experience. The threat of inhibition of self-expression and self-discovery may be inherent in instruction that is devoid of art, of fact devoid of fantasy. There is the spurious equation of scientific method with human experience, as described below.

> I spent all my younger life as a more or less orthodox amateur naturalist. As a pseudo-scientist, treating nature as some sort of intellectual puzzle or game, in which being able to name names and explain behaviourisms, to identify and understand machinery, constituted all the pleasures and the prizes. I became slowly aware of the inadequacy of this approach. That it insidiously cast nature as a kind of opponent, and the opposite team to be outwitted and beaten. That, in a number of very important ways it had distracted from the total experience and the total meaning of nature. Indeed, it exiled me from what I most needed to learn.
>
> (Fowles and Horvat, 1979)

This is similar to the destructive forces imposed on the medical students, and on the trainee psychiatrist. Similarly:

> What then are the objections to the use of the medical model? At worst it reduces man to the level of an 'it'. It takes no account of the richness of his inner world, his motives, conflicts and fantasies. It is the psychological component that makes psychiatry so very different from the rest of medicine and which the medically orientated, whether they be students or doctors, find so difficult to cope with.
>
> (Birtchnell, 1987)

And:

> Psychologically-minded school leavers select themselves out of medical school, for the prospect of a six year training in the medical sciences would not hold much appeal for them. Even if they did aspire eventually to become psychiatrists they may not be prepared to endure a non-psychological medical course in order to do so.
>
> (Birtchnell, 1987)

> The continuous exposure to critical situations reduces one's sensitivity to more trivial experiences, just as bright sunlight reduces one's awareness of delicate shades. A numbness settles in and as the callous attitude develops there is an inevitable drying up of finer feeling. One acquires a cold clinical indifference. This desensitization process tends to spread to other things like beauty, music and various forms of creativity and medical students become restricted in their interests.
>
> (Birtchnell, 1987)

During medical training, there are many everyday examples of the conversion of people into objects. Questioning of such incidents may be regarded as the subversive posturings of a flawed person. Similarly:

Part of the students' defensive reaction to their clinical experience is to focus exclusively on the patient's signs and symptoms and ignore, as far as possible, his emotional state. In their exposure to psychiatric patients, they are compelled to pay attention to that which hitherto they have been trying to avoid.

(Birtchnell, 1987)

Birtchnell has voiced sentiments which, if not overtly shared by other psychiatrists, lie dormant and seek expression. But by the time clinical indoctrination is complete, such reflections are often withered and vestigal.

The early selection of medical students predisposes them to an alienation from psychology and psychological approaches with the initial academic hurdle of GCSE 'A' levels in physics, chemistry and biology. The student is now established in his or her withdrawal from art and its capacity to elaborate on fundamental truths which are too subtle, intuitive and unverifiable for science to recognize or comprehend. A predisposition towards science is mainly conducted by professionals with a purely scientific bent, often research-orientated with tunnel vision for one scientific aspect of the person; usually physiologically or anatomically isolated from the whole, and denying the essential gestalt. This preoccupation with science is paradoxical, as psychiatry is notoriously unscientific, with an emphasis on implementation of techniques, rather than meeting the needs of the person. On balance, psychiatry may be closer to religion than science. In psychiatry, the curriculum (and assessment) has been largely dictated by those physicians firmly ensconced within the upper echelons of the hierarchy of medicine, clinging tenaciously to their medical credentials, and with a vested interest in retaining psychiatry within the medical model.

The family origins of many psychiatrists will have incorporated behavioural codes which demanded conformity and obedience to the dictums of the group. Most creative people, however, show early evidence of group deviance in their defiance of established codes, their questioning of ritual patterns, and a disregard for the approbation of the tribal elders. The early unquestioning acceptance of rules, and the imprinting of group identity militates against the logical reasoning of ethical dilemmas and the need to do so.

Those persons most appropriate to a specialization in psychiatry, therefore, will find the medical curriculum arduous, frustrating and inhibiting, while simultaneously denying them the capacity for personal growth. Conversely, the student adapting readily to the medical curriculum will find essential psychiatric concepts and modes of thinking difficult both to absorb and to practise. The scenario, therefore, is set for conflict, hostility and a process which obstructs the selection and training of those people most suited to provide an appropriate service within the mental health orbit. These are generalizations; some psychiatrists will have survived, with keener perceptions borne of stress. But what strange ignoble alchemy has produced this irony? Sadly, the answer lies in human aspirations, motivated by the need for power and status, as opposed to service. Such a destructive system is self-perpetuating, and effective intervention has been assiduously aborted.

CROSS-CULTURAL ASPECTS

Rowe (1983) has commented on the psychiatrist from another culture:

> Perhaps your good psychiatrist may decide to hold no more than a watching brief over you and arrange for you to see his junior doctor. You may have to make some adjustments to your own way of thinking and speaking when you are with your junior doctor since in the UK now a great many of the junior posts in psychiatry are held by doctors for whom English is not their first language or, even if it is, come from countries very different from Britain. Such men (and a few women) are usually devoted and hard working doctors, but they are at a disadvantage in a medical speciality which relies on language and an intimate knowledge of the society from which the patient comes. The diagnosis of depression depends so much on cultural values. If endogenous depression means a depression for which no cause in the patient's life can be found, and if the doctor doing the diagnosing believes that all a woman needs to make her happy is a husband, a home and children, then a depressed married woman is likely to be diagnosed as having endogenous depression and treated accordingly, which means a great likelihood of receiving only drugs and ECT and little psychotherapy.

These elements of selection and training, together with the preponderance of foreign graduates in psychiatry, have accentuated the organic aspects of psychiatry which have gained precedence, status and general dominance in the UK. This has been at the expense of psychotherapeutic techniques, and is reflected not only in the major psychiatric journals and literature, but also in the qualifying examination for membership of the Royal College of Psychiatrists. The bulk of factual information to be elicited by multiple choice questions and the number of specialized science areas. The ability to communicate (and a capacity to deal with ambiguity) reveal the lack of credence given to those areas of skill which many people might regard as essential. This is the area of constructive feeling in the professional which enables clients to reveal their innermost experiences, to share them, to have them examined and understood as a precursor to therapy.

LISTENING SKILLS

Psychiatrists should study more generally (and more carefully) aspects of listening which are not just hearing, but conducted with an intensity divorced from an academic stereotype (with its preoccupation for collection of relevant data) and move on to the more exciting, but demanding, challenge of 'liberating feeling'. It is the exploration of feeling which is the vital essential ingredient of proper understanding. Only then is it possible to allow the clients the opportunity of understanding the reasons for their reactions or behaviour and of those around them. The professional may then begin to recognize his or her own self — sometimes with a painful clarity. The provision of an anodyne with tranquillizers or unctuous platitudes produces superficial and destructive goals.

The medical graduate, and therefore the consultant psychiatrist, will have lived a comparatively aesthetically impoverished existence because of the demands of the profession. He or she will leave school with the requisite science GCSEs, so that the vulnerable years of maturity of late adolescence have evaporated, denying contact with humanities subjects. At medical school, anatomy and physiology and associated sciences force the student into thinking of the parts, and not the whole. Indeed, he or she cannot afford the luxury of contemplative, creative thinking, because such a vast array of facts must be accumulated for regurgitation to satisfy the examiners that this mental set demands a particular discipline. By the time clinical contact is made with the whole person, the student is already programmed to dissect and analyse the parts via isolation of the bits from the whole.

Eventually, such students will qualify with the prefix 'Doctor' and with the expectations from others that this title bestows. They may be well aware of this falsity of competence and bravely attempt to allay their fears. They may live the role demanded by expectations, and recognize the necessity to accumulate facts whilst already programmed to exclude the intrusion of 'non-professional' thoughts which should have included questions about themselves, as well as those around them, within a philosophical context. Certainly they have power — a particularly dangerous commodity when associated with assumed grandiosity.

Of course there are survivors:

When I started in general practice fifteen years ago I was a little dismayed to discover that most of my patients were not ill at all, at least not in the way hospital patients were ill. Even when I could not do anything people wanted to talk to me and seemed to appreciate having me around to listen to them. Over the years I came to know these people better and my affection (for most of them) increased. Naturally there were problems arising from such close contact with other people's emotions. Many patients made me feel angry or upset and to some I behaved badly. Normally I was there to share the patient's feelings and take an interest. It was, and I hope remains, a person-centred style of medicine in which disease control and disease prevention have an important place but are never allowed to degrade the patient into a mere object of the doctor's activities. The problem is that the frame of mind required for ticking off a mental check list or launching opportunistic health education sorties is quite different from the frame of mind required to listen to someone talking about a problem. This is especially so if the problem is a painful one or it lies concealed in a tangle of ambiguous feelings and physical sensations. For that you need to be able to forget your check lists and your questions; your mind almost needs to be a complete blank so that you can tune into your patient's moods.

(BMJ, 1988)

Jones (1978) has noted how psychiatry has been pulled into the organization, structures and professional modes of general medicine. It has thus become a medical specialism, a small part of general medicine. An insidious drift into veterinary psychiatry may allow people to enter hospital with the most complex and appalling problems, be given their pills and their ECT, and go out again to those same problems without ever having had a chance to discuss with anyone what was wrong. Jones has provided a critical analysis of psychiatry in practice, from a person in another discipline. Such clarity and wisdom identified the source of many ethical problems, with constructive and compassionate pointers towards solutions.

Storr (1983) has noted:

Years ago, when I was training at the Maudsley Hospital, we were taught that there are two kinds of depression, reactive and endogenous. I am glad to say that I never accepted the validity of this distinction. All it seemed to mean was that, in cases labelled reactive the doctor could define an obvious external cause for depression, like bereavement or bankruptcy, which he could see might cause depression in himself. Where no such obvious circumstances could be discerned the doctor concealed his ignorance by calling the patient's condition 'endogenous'. The word endogenous ought to be forbidden in psychiatry. Its implication that the condition so described is rooted in the patient's genetic structure discourages research. Much the same stricture is applied to the use of the phrase 'depressive illness' or 'affective disorder'. The assumptions underlying this use of language have prevented us from understanding depression. Depression is not an illness which one catches like influenza but a psychobiological reaction which can be provoked in any of us given appropriate circumstances, and which may have some positive uses.

A fundamental precept for an ethical approach to be adopted by therapists in their relationships with clients was identified. 'The therapist's repeated acceptance of, tolerance of, and dare I say, love for, the patient gradually allows his incorporation into the patient's inner world so that he continues to exist even when the patient is no longer seeing him'

(Storr, 1983).

A PARALLEL EXAMPLE

Several features of the psychiatrist's background might contribute to a failure of ethical awareness. Nurses also may be confronted by incidents found to be unacceptable with resulting conflicts and dilemmas under threatening circumstances. A parallel set of circumstances and associated problems confronted staff at Rampton Special Hospital in the late 1970s. That parallel situation clearly illustrates the degree of moral impoverishment within the mental health service and the implications for those staff members inclined to comment or intrude.

Included in a review of conditions at Rampton, published in November 1980, were 205 recommendations (Boynton, 1980). Undoubtedly the most important of the recommendations (and essential to the underlying purpose of the document) was the appointment of a Review Board for a three-year period specifically charged with the responsibility of ensuring that the proposals in the original report were instituted. Almost a decade later both the public and the profession remain largely uninformed. The relevance of that review to the ethos of other Special Hospitals has not been clearly enunciated nor acted upon.

The poignancy of the plight of the inmates of Rampton may have been eroded by time — an erosion was enhanced by the bland verbiage of the 'Boynton Report'. This report partly concealed and partly camouflaged the unacceptable, and sometimes criminal, practices perpetrated for over a decade under the auspices of the Department of Health. Following the showing of the Yorkshire Television film *The Secret Hospital* in May 1979, and after a brief period of public agonizing, apprehension was allayed (and the momentum for active intervention was soon enmeshed) in enquiries by the police and by the appointment of the Boynton Review Committee. Following publication of the report of the review of Rampton Hospital, a public confession from these authorities responsible for the situation might optimistically have been anticipated. As a preliminary to an overall reappraisal with appropriate corrective measures in all branches of the service, the revelations contained a specific use.

The reaction of the medical hierarchy to exposures within its responsibility was diffident and muted, if not altogether absent. An editorial in the Lancet (1980) however, stated that:

The Boynton Committee have produced a long list of unsatisfactory features, including a penal atmosphere, a patient population that is too large, a lack of professional leadership, the dominance of the Prison Officers' Association, a nurse shift system which confines patients to their rooms for 11 hours and an excessive number of patients awaiting transfer', and later: 'whether or not the Boynton Report is implemented, and whether or not in 12 months there will always remain one embarrassing, conscience pricking question for the medical profession. How is it that it takes a muck-raking television programme to uncover the horrors of yet another British mental hospital? Where was the Royal College of Psychiatrists?

An editorial in World Medicine (1980) made a similar observation:

'And why did it take a commercial television company, with MIND backing it up in the rear, rather than leaders of the psychiatric, nursing and social work professions, to reveal to a horrified world what was happening?'

Despite the dry, measured, rather aggrieved tone of the Boynton Report, which tended to obscure the enormity of the indictment it contained, one small aspect of that report indicated the implications of the underlying regime and its attendant brutalization of staff and inmates.

When talking of the daily life of inmates at Rampton, there seemed to be some crack in the wall of cold objectivity which characterized most of the report via a glimpse of the 'therapeutic' day. It became clear that inmates slept in cell-like side rooms and dormitories, containing no furniture except beds. After inmates were unlocked from their rooms in the morning, beds were stripped and searched. The inmates then proceeded in single file to the sluice with their chamber pots. After collecting day clothes they went to the main corridor or the billiard room, where they stood together to dress. After cleaning beds and bedrooms they loitered outside awaiting inspection. If passed, they were ordered to empty their buckets. There was no further access to their rooms for the rest of the day. Then they queued for the washroom. There was little talking, but a great sense of urgency. One 'kitchen man' brought all the nurses tea as they stood observing the inmates dress. Before breakfast inmates formed a queue in the main corridor and were counted. They showed their locker keys to the duty nurse to prove that they had not been lost. At meal times, in most maximum security wards, there was silence. Bread was given out by a nurse by hand straight from the bag. After breakfast inmates formed a queue and were counted again. Inmates in one ward would scrub floors and wash down walls throughout the morning. At midday inmates queued for a rub-down search. No-one could go to their rooms; in any case there were no personal possessions. After lunch they sat in the day/TV room which had chairs in rows and some occasional tables for letter writing or playing cards. Most nurses sat along the wall talking to each other, watching TV, reading newspapers. If an inmate wanted to light a cigarette he or she had to ask one of the nurses for permission to do so. Having lit the cigarette in the corridor, the inmate had to wait on the threshold saying: 'Please can I come in sir?'

With such an overt exposure of the hospital ethos, which even the fastidious Boynton Report was unable to obscure, the implications of subtle and covert damage are horrifying. Obvious questions which arise logically from such observations were not asked, leaving those with ulti-mate responsibility free from culpability. The multiplicity of superficial (and sometimes irrelevant) questions which were raised served to obscure the fundamental conclusion that Rampton was impossible to disguise as a hospital with all its distorting superstructure of expensive 'professional' input. It was, in fact, a prison, devoid of the monitoring, scrutiny and concern correctly accorded to criminal populations within the penal system.

Under the guise of a 'special hospital' there was an inbred, self-perpetua-ting, self-protective institution, which was a model of Goffman's clear denunciation of such establishments. It was rigid, impenetrable and crip-pling to staff and inmates. The Boynton Report, constructed in the 18 months following the television penetration of Rampton also included such revealing comments as: 'we were pleased to learn that since we have been working at Rampton a committee has been set up' (Boynton, 1980).

A PERSONAL EXPERIENCE

Within three months of arrival at Rampton (a maximum security hospital in Nottinghamshire, UK) in June 1978 and, unaware of the forthcoming television production, my misgivings were made absolutely clear in strong-worded depositions, and verbally, on numerous occasions to senior doc-tors and administrators in the DHSS. A subsequent publication (Inskip and Edwards, 1979) stated: 'many enquiries could have been prevented if warning signs had not been ignored and decisive action had been taken earlier', and again: 'on occasions when doctors or other professional col-leagues decide that they are unable to provide the minimum acceptable standard for some aspects of care they should make it plain in writing to the appropriate authority and insist on a written answer on how the gap is to be filled'.

Within a few weeks of my arrival at Rampton it became obvious that it was impossible to function effectively as a consultant in psychiatry. It was not the practice to interview inmates in privacy, unaccompanied by nurs-ing staff, and there was little sign of conventional doctor/client relationship. Requests to see inmates alone were countered by arguments that this was both impracticable and unnecessary.

Inmates were admitted by the DHSS without consultation with the receiving psychiatrist. It seemed that the expectations nursing staff had of the consultant was of someone who prescribed medication when so prompted, and endorsed methods of control such as seclusion, the imposition of penalties and loss of privileges. Case conferences, first introduced in 1976, gave little indication of a considered plan of rehabilitation, but rather an account of behaviour which would either justify or debarr a person from movement within the hospital system. What appeared to be missing was any evaluation by professional staff as to why the person was disturbed and what methods of treatment would be available to a multi-disciplinary team to cope with periods of disturbance.

There was a sad poignancy in that clients with a mental handicap (the largest category at Rampton) were the least able to conform to such a system, and were more prone to express frustration or distress through physical acts of aggression. Often these individuals did not possess the verbal or social skills necessary to deal with such feelings in an acceptable manner. Inevitably, the resulting altercations would result in a very slow passage through the system. One saw that this system tended to induce dependence on staff, and an increasing inability to cope with the pressures of life outside an institutional setting. So, the obvious question arose: 'How could one intrude effectively on such a situation?'

Letters were sent to the appropriate administrative authorities, stating that medical coverage for the physical care of inmates was inadequate and constituted a serious hazard. No acknowledgement was ever received. A subsequent letter sent to the Permanent Secretary of the DHSS met with an acknowledgement and the promise of future discussion.

In addition to the 'Elliott Report' (completed and submitted to the Department in 1974) there had been another report which preceeded it. Both reports had stated very clearly what the Boynton Report subsequently reiterated. The recommendations for transferring a stagnant custodial institution into a therapeutic rehabilitative hospital had been treated with the apathy and ineptitude which was characteristic of the dealings of the Department of Health with its largest special hospital.

A comprehensive document was submitted to the Department, suggesting that to intrude successfully on the present situation would require the introduction of other treatment modalities, staff training, frequent case conferences and a gradual re-orientation of attitudes. The submission was that any change should rely on the quality and quantity of medical staff and that until such time as staffing did improve, people were existing in an in-built, self-perpetuating system of destructive forces. Again, no acknowledgement or response was forthcoming. The simple objective was to acquire acceptable basic standards.

Six months after my arrival at Rampton I was joined by a consultant who allied himself to this goal. Fifteen months later that colleague resigned, humiliated and disillusioned. He (correctly) feared for his professional future if he continued to battle against overwhelming odds, devoid of any support from professional bodies. Indeed he joined me in resort to medical defence societies to guard against the depredations provoked by our questioning of the system. It was our impression that our consultant colleagues condoned and supported the system we decried — a conclusion reinforced by their previous failure to intervene. Such attitudes in consultant psychiatric staff can exist and survive and apparently recruit rewards. On this point Boynton (1980) made the following comment:

> They [the consultants] rejected any suggestion that the doctors individually or corporately had a role to play in the way the hospital was run or the philosophies of treatment which should be adopted. Some appointments are made on the grounds of expediency rather than suitability.

The Royal College of Psychiatrists continued to condone the appointment of physicians, without a basic qualification in psychiatry, to long-term locum consultant posts in psychiatry at Rampton.

Familiarity with events within the hospital in the months preceding the Yorkshire Television programme (*The Secret Hospital*, shown in May 1979) might have given adequate warning, and provided an indicator of anticipated staff reaction. The nurses, with the support and encouragement of their union (the Prison Officers' Association) had pursued the only possible method of care available, within the limitations imposed by their experience and training, and in the absence of medical leadership. Specifically, this was control by means of medication and a rigid, uncompromising regime.

At times of threat, groups inevitably heed the strident, aggressive and militant voices amongst them, because they articulate group anger and group fear. The problems underlying these reactions tend to be compounded. There are also destructive voices in all grades of staff within such an institution, ready to foster such views and use them for their own purposes. The result is usually insularity, denial, self-justification and stubborness, with abandonment of conciliation and reason. Under such circumstances, those who suffer must inevitably be the inmates.

Some conclusions regarding the Rampton affair were:

1. No change would have been implemented at Rampton had it not been for the television programme which was shown in May 1979.
2. It is impossible for an individual doctor to initiate change unless support is recruited from appropriate medical organizations. While MIND had

provided guidance and support, the BMA and the Royal College of
Psychiatrists had remained aloof.
3. The DHSS had failed in its function of management. The Department's
   behaviour was characterized by apathy and ineptitude, both clinically
   and managerially, placing expediency before principle.
4. The nurses at Rampton Hospital had been scapegoated, and bore the
   full thrust of criticism for inadequacies in areas other than their own.
5. Conditions in Rampton constituted a cynical deprivation of the basic
   human rights.

These conclusions were, in part, endorsed in an article by a member of
staff at Rampton (Baldwin, 1984), who wrote:

> Rampton contains some excellent staff whose skills, work records,
> expertise and experience are second to none. Owing to poor manage-
> ment selection and inadequate screening, however, deviant staff have
> been appointed despite their rejection by other health service pro-
> fessionals. This tendency to appoint people with insufficient qualifi-
> cations and expertise has resulted in a subsequent devaluation of the
> service provided and of the clients themselves. Surrounding deviant
> clients with deviant workers becomes a recipe for inadequate socialis-
> ation. The very presence of emotionally unstable individuals in key staff
> roles in the institution has worsened the subtle effects of institutionalis-
> ation. It is now necessary, therefore, to screen out those individuals
> who are displaying bizarre mannerisms or who are beset with verbal
> and non-verbal communication problems. In an environment where
> understanding of clients requires knowledge about human relation-
> ships, it is tragic that a percentage of key medical staff do not possess
> linguistic skills.

Baldwin (1984) states later that:

> The system has violated personal rights and freedoms in the name
> of rehabilitation. Fundamental personal choices are often denied for
> administrative convenience.

Five years after the Boynton Report, it appeared that progress had been
engulfed by the deceptive verbiage which characterized the meanderings
of a multiplicity of committees. As one writer (*Hospital Doctor*, 1985)
observed, an independent enquiry into the care of inmates in maximum
security hospitals had been deferred indefinitely, and may not take place
at all. The wheels of a dithering beaurocracy continued to trundle around,
rather than towards, the problem. In sum, there had been a continuing
failure to address the appropriate professionals to the basic task of providing expertise and action to a group who were disadvantaged and inarticu-

late. This was an unsatisfactory conclusion to an ethical disaster in which psychiatry in the UK should be regarded as culpable.

The foregoing comments have been critical. In mitigation, it should be stated that there are further ethical components which bring unacceptable pressures on special hospitals. These include the failure of the penal system to cope with the 'mentally abnormal' offender, and the reluctance of consultant psychiatrists in conventional mental hospitals to accept such individuals as patients. In this, they are aided and abetted by such dubious ideals as conservation of the 'open door policy' and 'the therapeutic community'. Such attitudes have received the support of the powerful nursing unions in mental hospitals, and there has been an inevitable loss of expertise in these institutions in dealing with the problem. This has been combined with the apprehension of staff in coping with inmates whose condition is outside their experience or training. Special hospitals share with regional secure units and prisons the powerful and enduring tendency of society to isolate and ignore the 'mentally abnormal offender', while expurgating their guilt with orchestrated criticisms of individuals who work in such institutions when they are seen to be imperfect in their attempts to cope with this problem. Finally a lack of political commitment exists in an area which carries little political mileage.

ETHICS IN FORENSIC PSYCHIATRY

There is a problem relating to physicians who feel themselves under pressure to categorize and treat. Psychiatrists can seldom afford the luxury of a philosophical, contemplative approach incorporating sociological, linguistic and theological ingredients, when confronted with the reality of their situation. This was described by Kubie (1971), claiming that there is one setting in which it is impossible for the student of psychiatry to become a psychiatrist:

> This is the setting which uses only an assembly-line approach to patients and where the official attitude is to scorn sustained individual interaction and to take pride in brief interviews and rapid turnover.

In the same article, Kubie states:

> Mention has already been made of the limitations on psychiatric skills which result from total acceptance of one ideology/one type of explanation for mental illness. There is the serious hazard for patients which occasionally arises from this when the psychiatrist is intensely motivated to cure at all costs, when he has the passionate and excessive zeal to treat and an unfortunate inability to accept that in the present state of knowledge we are not infrequently therapeutically impotent. Out of this attitude have come some of the abuses of psychiatry, the excessive use

of ECT, multiple leucotomy operations, excessive use of drugs, and worst of all the use of legal methods of restraint which under the Mental Health Act allow the psychiatrist, acting of course honestly although ignorantly, to impose excessive treatment.

Kubie identifies one of the causes for this situation. When the blueprint for the mental health services was drawn up in 1971, it was based upon several propositions whose only claim was that they suited the limited human and financial resources of the country at the time. The psychological element in mental illness, as something which the psychiatrist's training might equip him or her to understand, and for which treatment might be advisable, was ignored altogether. Indeed, no provision was made initially in the mental health services for psychologists or psychotherapists. This theme was again emphasized by Jones (1978):

> In practice, psychiatry was increasingly pulled into the organisations, the structures and the professional models of general medicine. It has become a medical specialism, a small part of general medicine. There was a moment in time when it might have been much more.

THE WIDER PROBLEMS

The road ahead is difficult. Many ethical and educational problems within the medical model lie in the hands of the General Medical Council.

> The GMC is too large; its staff are overloaded, its powers too concentrated, and its communications poor. The Council's many internal problems often seem to occupy members of the Council and staff more than the pressing problems of improving education and competence and being seen to serve the public interest. In many ways it seems like an old-fashioned body that resents the modern world.
>
> (Smith, 1989)

Similarly:

> I have argued that, today, the notion of a person 'having a mental illness' is scientifically crippling. It provides professional assent to a popular rationalisation, namely, the problems of living experienced and expressed in terms of so called psychiatric symptoms are basically similar to bodily diseases. Moreover, the concept of mental illness also undermines the principle of personal responsibility, the ground on which all free political institutions rest. For the individual, the notion of mental illness precludes an enquiring attitude towards his conflicts which his 'symptoms' at once conceal and reveal. For a society it precludes regarding individuals as responsible persons, inviting, instead, the treatment of them as irresponsible patients. Although powerful institutional forces

lend their massive weight to the tradition of keeping psychiatric problems within the conceptual framework of medicine, the moral and scientific challenge is clear; we must recast and redefine the problem of 'mental illness' so that it may be encompassed in a morally explicit science of man.

(Szasz, 1962)

A technological civilization has developed; medicine has been conspicuously tardy when deliberating on the effects of this rapid change on the mind and the body. Ethical considerations are more important in direct proportion to technological advances. With the acquisition of knowledge in any sphere an overview, prior to re-assessment, is required. This is particularly relevant to scientists who, enamoured of their discoveries in some narrow field, stray into areas which transcend their legitimate boundaries. As with the geneticist requiring strictures and limitations and ethical guidance, so psychiatrists require the observations, controls and ethical principles derived from disparate sources of knowledge. Only then can comprehensive and fruitful analysis of the contribution from psychiatry be incorporated within mental health services on a sound ethical basis. And only by so doing will clients receive the attention which derives from wisdom and compassion.

There are large areas of psychiatry which at present demand conventional medical input in the form of physical methods of treatment for recognized and established diagnostic entities. Attempts to ameliorate psychotic states and behaviour must, however, recruit the involvement of all disciplines. Intervention with people who are psychotic is not the sole province of psychiatrists. In addition, disorders which arise directly from neurological damage will derive initial benefit from strictly medical intervention but subsequent management will again rely on an inter-disciplinary approach.

Resistance is required against being drawn into any debate which rests on a confrontation between genetics and environment as dominant in the production of mental disorder. There is some evidence of a genetic component in the development of psychotic states; physical methods of treatment, including drug therapies, have sometimes proved effective in the control of psychotic symptoms. Seriously disturbed persons have been relieved of those elements which distort and remove them from reality via medication. Thereafter, psychotherapy should be used to maintain and improve mental health. A thorough analysis of the control concept indicates that a psychosocial approach should complement physical treatments.

Mental health team workers who have been fortunate enough to work in units enjoying the luxury of low staff/client ratios, where the unit philosophy is based on the reduction of fear, avoidance of humiliation and the enhancement of self-worth., find their therapeutic response to be profoundly affected. For clients who have infringed the rights of others, and whose disturbed behaviour has included the partial or complete destruction of their victims, a therapeutic milieu is essential with restrictions and corrective training. The primary ingredient remains the provision of an environment (albeit protective of clients and public) which allows remorse, whilst fostering nobility. This is a difficult therapeutic amalgam, which is impossible to realize in the understaffed, conventional setting lacking common goals, interdisciplinary cohesion and the rewards of intimacy and continuity in client care.

An attempt at exploration of the congruity of aesthetic awareness and empathy has been made, with particular reference to the implications and use of language in psychiatry. The point here is not to debate the relevance or otherwise of works on theology and philosophy to clinical practice. Rather, such works stimulate questioning, re-appraisal and (if the recipient has a fertile mind — knowing how little they know) learning may occur in areas not incorporated into a training curriculum. It is necessary to find escape routes from the confines of a restricted lifestyle, and it need not be in esoteric areas, but from the liberation inherent in any form of creativity.

A familiar method of reinforcing group solidarity is through rituals and ceremony, rewarding those who respond with sycophancy and conformity. In the Merit Award system, this is done with gifts of money. These generous donations are given secretly under the guise of recognition of exceptional contribution to the speciality and, by implication, to the care of clients. Despite sustained criticisms this unacceptable practice continues. Even the most hardened potentate in the psychiatric hierarchy must appreciate the ethical nihilism in such a concept, and its potentiation of values alien to an acceptable moral framework for any vocation but inimical to psychiatry.

Patronage has been incorporated in the criteria for receipt of fellowships and memberships of the Royal College of Psychiatrists. On the inception of the Royal College, 'goodies' were distributed to conforming members in the granting of memberships and fellowships. The absurdity and intrinsic damage of this distribution of largesse was revealed in the discovery that even fellowships of the Royal College of Psychiatry could be gained without having sat or trained for basic psychiatric qualifications.

This exposure of the supremacy of power over principle, as a motivating factor in a speciality which is prepared to make authoritarian statements on moral determinants, has an obvious irony. Expediency and morality are incompatible; this disparity had an added component of contrivance and self-interest (which militates against the provision of an appropriate service in the mental health area). Psychiatrists have strayed into dangerous country, but have done so with zeal and enthusiasm. Physicians, like some other health professionals, have seized power to obtain financial, material and professional privilege. Whilst this may be 'dangerous country', it has been enthusiastically explored. A secrecy which solidifies the establishment and is conducive to rigidity, insularity and rejection of self-appraisal is not the kind of club which will recruit members with any degree of integrity. It will be a club fearful of creativity and individuality. It will perpetuate and reinforce all that is bad, obscuring any clear perceptions of the true role of the psychiatrist, and opposed to its more worthy aspirations.

It is not necessary to enumerate and identify the persistent failures and abuses in British psychiatry. Those outside the profession have done this service; not least those damaged clients, whose voices are being heard clearly, with their numbing exposure of the degradation to which they have been subjected. There is poignancy and validity to their accounts, endorsed by the muted factual recounting of the process of their own destruction, and then the occasional denoument in which those responsible are understood and forgiven.

Acquaintance with the sociological implications of professionalism provides safeguards against the abuse of power. A knowledge of the sociological habitat in which an individual resides should determine the superstructure of ethical codes. In short, a grounding in sociology should take precedence, in the training of a psychiatrist, over the niceties of neuronal transmission. Such a widening of horizons will prove salutory and initiate questioning. School teachers should be the most valued professionals, for it is the children who must be given the tools to structure appropriate ethical concepts and the moral integrity to challenge destructive professional precepts. Until then, the occasional tilt at the windmills of established psychiatry in the UK will potentiate martyrdom, rather than maturity.

Emancipation involves not only respect and affection and understanding for those in care but for fellow team mates in the mental health services. Such is the nature of the service professionals attempt to provide that they require the succour and the guidance of each other. It is a demanding and at times exsanguinating vocation, which renders professionals vulnerable to criticism and to cynicism. The objective in health services is the transfer to clients of the tools for their own recovery, and to give them the credit for any benefit which might accrue. Professionals should eschew dependency and try to avoid the feeding of their own narcissism. They are exposed often to loneliness, insecurity and fear. In order to maintain enlightened, ethical conduct they require supportive intimacy and compassionate understanding of other workers in all disciplines. This can only be achieved by an awareness arising from interdisciplinary dialogue and the incorporation in training of familiarity with these disciplines. By doing so, a platform is provided for the questioning unison for growth and the protection of clients.

In addressing the subject of ethics and psychiatry, professionals face those questions whose answers will facilitate an enlightenment which will assist in preventing further damage to clients. The answers will not be found in the imposition of rules, regulations, prohibitions and penalties for inappropriate behaviour, but rather in a distancing from the restricting ethos of medicine, and the acquisition of sociological, philosophical and psychological truths which allow creative analysis at the expense of technological tunnel vision.

The mental health disciplines are largely science-based and science-dominated. This has been, and remains, a firm foundation for the service, ensuring those safeguards equate with validation, factual confirmation and knowledge of the components of the focus of concern. The mind, however, does not easily lend itself to revelation within the confines of science. To engage, explore and understand its ramifications, professionals must incorporate those branches of knowledge concerned with humankind and culture.

It is unproductive to continue to argue the case for ethical reform within psychiatry by providing goals, guidelines, penalties and formulations. What is required is radical change of a fundamental nature: not cosmetic improvement; not window dressing. Rather, as should have occurred at Rampton following its exposure, a more drastic intervention is required incorporating a concept which considers medicine as a sub-speciality of the social sciences. Psychiatry should become a subsidiary of psychology and those people wishing to practise within the mental health service should have a training in which medicine plays a subordinate role. This would select those people more likely to comprehend the implications of the vocation and the needs of clients, while at the same time providing a platform for constructive consideration of ethical issues in mental health care.

CONCLUSIONS

One possible conclusion is that psychiatry should be restructured as a psychological, not medical discipline. This presumes, however, that psychiatry is presently a medical discipline; many critics have argued that psychiatry has the guise of medicine, but is rather a means of social control. Certainly, within the 'medical hierarchy', psychiatry is at the bottom of the professional pile. Some of the sternest critics of psychiatrists have been other physicians.

It is suggested that the correct code of ethics will evolve from those precepts we develop for ourselves. Such precepts are born of attempts to deal with pain and perceptions, and the search for a true understanding of ourselves will give us courage and the necessity to identify and defend the rights of those in our care.

When the causes of malpractice have been examined, guidelines given, penalties clarified, codes promulgated and exhortations heeded, it will still remain with the individual worker to exercise his or her own moral philosophy. No jurisdiction will protect our clients. In the final analysis appropriate ethical behaviour will depend on the respect, the understanding and the concern we have for others.

REFERENCES

Baldwin, S. (1984) Unacceptable Practices. *Community Care*, 1st March, 21–6.

Birtchnell, J. (1987) A psychiatrist speaks out. *British Journal of Clinical and Social Psychiatry*, 5(2), 223–5.

BMJ (1988) Editorial. *British Medical Journal*, **296**, 1198.

Boynton, J. (1980) *The Report of the Committee of Investigation at Rampton Hospital*, HMSO, London.

Cambell, A. V. (1976) *Moral Dilemmas in Medicine*. Churchill Livingstone, London.

Fowles, J. and Horvat, F. (1979) *The Tree*. Auram Press, London.

Goffman, E. (1961) *Asylums*. Penguin, Harmondsworth.

Hospital Doctor (1985) Security patient probe put on ice. 7th February, 571.

Inskip, J. H. and Edwards, J. G. (1979) Mental hospital enquiries. *Lancet*, 658–60.

Jones, K. (1978) Society looks at the psychiatrist. *British Journal of Psychiatry*, **132**, 321–332.

Kubie, I. S. (1971) Retreat from patients. *Archives of General Psychiatry*, **24**, 98–106.

Laing, R. D. (1967) *The Politics of Experience and the Bird of Paradise*. Penguin, London.

Lancet (1980) Editorial. Close Rampton? **8205**, 1171–2.

Rowe, D. (1983) *Depression: The Way out of your Prison*. Fontana, London.

Smith, R. (1989) Profile of the GMC. *British Medical Journal*, **299**, 40.

Storr, A (1983) A psychotherapist looks at depression. *British Journal of Psychiatry*, **143**, 431–435.

Szasz, T. S. (1974) *The Myth of Mental Illness*. Harper and Row, New York.

World Medicine (1980) Editorial. November 29, 5.

Chapter Five

Ethical issues in work with older people

CHRISTINE BARROWCLOUGH AND IAN FLEMING

EDITORS' INTRODUCTION

People who need help to live their lives may be handicapped physically, or may have difficulty dealing with the dilemmas posed by ordinary life. Older people can experience both of these handicaps and may also be handicapped by the negative views of a society obsessed with youth, health and vigour. Older people can experience difficulty in overcoming these obstacles without extra help. Paradoxically, many older people may be conditioned to such an extent that they feel unworthy of the very help which they so badly need. Furthermore, a second-generational handicap can also exist: some older people feel that such help is no more than 'charity' and, as such, should be rejected.

In this chapter **Christine Barrowclough** and **Ian Fleming** discuss the difficulties experienced by older people and the dilemmas, faced by service providers, in deciding how, exactly, to provide for their needs.

Ethical issues in work with older people

Those persons involved in health care and social service systems will be aware of the demographic statistics which have highlighted the increasing proportion of older people in the population. The future needs of these old and very old people will be of concern to all 'caring' professions, and the number of posts for workers who will specialize in providing a service to older people has increased. Such posts are often not popular but in recent years there has been a growth of interest in the nature of services for older people. Moral and ethical issues need to be examined, since there are some important reasons why older people are particularly vulnerable to having their rights violated. These include: the high incidence of physical and mental disability in very old people; the fact that they are more likely to be institutionalized than younger people; and the negative image of old age which predominates in Western culture.

A number of writers have recently advised of the faulty thinking inherent in theories and practice, whereby dependency is viewed as a function of old age. O'Donohue *et al.* (1986) have reminded behaviour analysts that the central tenets of behaviourism enable behaviour therapists to reject the developmental view of an older person's behaviour where age is used as an explanatory entity. Social scientists have defined older people clearly as a socially-determined group, whose dependency has been socially manufactured (Phillipson and Walker, 1986); and service agents have been urged to take this into account when planning interventions (Walker, 1983).

Despite these attempts to urge practitioners to view older clients as people whose behaviour is as much shaped by their environment, and by social and economic constraints, as by biological consequences of getting older, we are required to work in a culture which does not value its older people and whose social depreciation is reflected in inadequate services which may only enhance the dependent status of its recipients. This 'ageism' has a pervasive influence in services for older people and, as workers within that system, it is sometimes difficult to maintain a non-ageist stance and give a good service to the client.

Norman (1986) provided examples of ageism at work in health and social services but unfortunately failed to suggest any reason for its potency. Simone de Beauvoir, in her worldly book *Old Age* attempted to do this. Her examination of old age, in both past and present, gathers an enormous breadth of data from anthropology, ethology, sociology, psychology and history. She sees the attitudes of a particular society towards its old people as being neither static, nor predetermined, but instead closely related to the political priorities of that society. 'This status depends upon the aims the country sets itself . . . it is the meaning that men attribute to their life, it is their entire system of values that define the meaning of old age. The reverse applies: by the way in which a society behaves towards its old people, it uncovers the naked and, often carefully hidden, truth about its real principles and aims' (de Beauvoir, 1977).

Thus, de Beauvoir locates the prejudices of 'ageism' in the wider attitudes and behaviours of a particular society. Furthermore, she sees these as being largely determined by the culture of a particular society which, in turn, is shaped by its economic development and political organization. Prejudices about old age are connected fundamentally to ideas about power and a person's place in the productive process. Lack of productive power is deemed to be indicative of lack of value generally.

The economic devaluation of old people is also discussed by Walker (1983) in his analyses of social policy towards older people in Britain:

The exclusion of older workers from the labour market has formed the basis for a more general devaluation of the contribution and social status of older people in British society, a judgment which incidentally is denied by the contribution of older people to family relationships . . . This changing social relationship between the labour market has formed the basis for a more general spread of dependency amongst the elderly.

This chapter aims to look at some aspects of ageism within services for older people and aims to address some of the related difficulties and dilemmas faced by service agents.

ETHICAL PRINCIPLES

A fundamental problem which workers frequently face is how to balance the older person's needs for care and protection against the potential danger of overruling preferences or treating them as children (see Age Concern, 1986, for a full discussion of the legal aspects). This dilemma is made more complex by the frequent failure of services to offer care and protection which is not synonomous with custodial care; along with all the detrimental effects associated with 'custodial' services. Thus, intervention may not only reduce self-determination, and infringe individual liberty, but also adversely affect the individual's well-being.

Three general principles have developed to inform medical and therapeutic practice. These have been referred to as:

1. the *Principle of Beneficence* — in which the intervention should only be carried out for the benefit of the individual concerned and can be summed up in the adage 'above all, do no harm';
2. the *Principle of Autonomy* — in which the person's power and self-determination is the primary consideration; and
3. the *Principle of Just Distribution* — which applies to the requirement that any one individual should have the same right to access to services as any other.

Cadow (1980) suggested that conflict can arise between the first two of these principles since Power of Autonomy included fundamental requirements that the recipient of service benefits, whereas the Principle of Beneficence assumes the waving of autonomy in favour of receiving benefit.

Cadow also suggests that these ethical principles are affected by views held about ageing and older people by the general public. She cites the broadly utilitarian view which states that older people are less valuable than younger persons because of their lesser contribution to general social goals, or the collective happiness, and indicates that this may survive in the rationale for the 'degree-of-benefit', whereby preference is allocated to people who will show the greater potential for response to an intervention or therapy. In this way, there is a principle of discrimination in favour of young people. This principle is often implicit in services for older people, as will be illustrated later.

DECISION-MAKING

It is sometimes difficult for those who are employed in services for older people to ensure the service recipient is the older client, and that the older person has a real say in the services received. Although this problem may be observed most clearly when the older person is unable to verbalize preferences, as in the case of a person with advanced dementia, there are many examples of the failure to solicit the opinions of verbally competent older people, about actions or decisions which may have important effects on their lives. Steinberg *et al.* (1986) give examples from American studies where medical treatment was denied to many elderly nursing home patients, and they note the absence of the person's own request not to be treated in a list of factors influencing decisions to withhold 'non-heroic' life-saving treatment.

The literature on behaviour therapists shows their failure to involve older clients in the choice of treatment goals. The target behaviours for older people have been determined largely by other (and particularly younger) people. This situation has changed very little in the past 15 years. In a recent survey of 'behavioural-gerontological' research, Mosher-Ashley (1987) concludes: 'Elderly participants, both institutionalized and living independently, were rarely consulted in the target behaviour to be modified, selection of procedures to be employed, or even the reinforcers to be employed. The passive role of the elderly in behavioural treatment procedures can also be seen in the scarcity of studies employing self-management techniques or other individuals (e.g. peers) in the intervention plan'.

O'Donohue *et al.* (1986) also reviewed the behavioural literature on work with older people and made the same conclusion. They found that the older person was significantly involved in the determination of treatment goals in only three out of 29 behavioural 'geriatric' studies reviewed. Typical target behaviours which were indicative of this determination of treatment by others were: participation in ward activities; correct use of eating utensils; and incontinence. The paper gives some telling examples of mismatch between client and experimenter treatment goals. For example, they cite the oft-quoted research by Peterson *et al.* (1977) which has been very influential in the design of seating arrangements in establishments for older people. Peterson describes how the people in the study disrupted the new arrangements that the experimenter made with the furniture, causing him to re-arrange the furniture early in the morning before the people arose. 'In this study, the elderly clients' preferences for particular furniture arrangements were not only ignored but systematically countermanded' (O'Donohue *et al.*, 1986).

Earlier discussion of ethical principles has focused on whether decisions are made on behalf of older people — if so, by whom? — and on 'informed consent'. Behavioural interventions have long been held to be powerful and open to possible abuse. (e.g. Zangwill, 1980), although there is ample evidence that this situation is not necessarily inherent in interventions derived from a functional analysis of behaviour (e.g. Skinner, 1983).

Krasner and Ullman (1973) propose that the concept of freedom has two components: lack of coercion and ability to choose. They point out that behavioural therapists can, and should, successfully increase the freedom of others by increasing their repertoire of 'environment-changing behaviours'. O'Donohue *et al.* (1986) cite Krasner's suggestion that behaviour therapy should enable clients to learn to control, influence or design their own environment, specifically in the area of behavioural geriatrics. In addition, reference is made to Bandura's advice that behavioural therapists must do things *with* people, rather than *for* them or *to* them. Suggestions are made for training elderly clients in ways to influence their environment so that they might be able to counter-control those in power, rather than training staff or carers in principles of behavioural management. An example would be that of responding to a referral from a home for older people by working with an individual to enable him or her to obtain a desired goal, instead of formulating an intervention to reduce or eliminate a 'problem behaviour'. Thus, instead of seeking to extinguish behaviours which are viewed as inappropriate (such as shouting out, or repeatedly asking for staff intervention) one would see the elderly person as the client and formulate with him or her a goal which would involve gaining more attention.

This approach has similarities with the constructional approach (Goldiamond, 1974; Fleming *et al.*, 1983) which aims to increase, rather than decrease, the range of behaviours available to the person. In particular, Goldiamond's view is that the therapeutic contract is between the person who is to bring change and the person who is to be the subject of the change. If a person seeks help with his or her elderly relative, the contract would facilitate changing the behaviour of the younger relative, rather than the older person.

Several factors work against older people and may result in having their views overlooked or, worse still, overruled. One is that the older person is rarely the person who seeks help. Instead, problems are identified by some other agent — often a relative or neighbour for older people who live in their own homes, or an officer of the institution for those residing in institutional care. Older people may have difficulty in making their choices known to the service, including the choice of 'no service'.

An older woman who lives alone may illustrate this. Her son becomes increasingly concerned that his mother does little housework or cooking, and receives messages from neighbours about her frequent calls to their houses, particularly in the late evening. He and his wife respond by spending more time at his mother's, doing her housework, shopping and cooking meals. His mother appears to do less and less for herself and the son and daughter-in-law feel an increasing burden, ultimately contacting the general practitioner and social services. The old lady sees neither her loss of domestic skill performance, nor the increased contact with her family as problems. As a service provider entering this situation, it is difficult to remember who is the client and to identify her needs and wishes which may well be incompatible with those of the family. For example, she may wish to *increase* her contact with family members and enjoy their concern. Should one assist the client to achieve these targets? In this case, it would be advocated that both the son's and mother's needs are considered, preferably with independent help for both people. The likelihood, however, is that the services emphasize the younger person's needs, without involving the older person in the decision-making process. Alternatively, there may be some attempt to persuade the older person of the difficulties her son faces as a consequence of her behaviour. This tendency by younger people to view their own lives and those of their younger friends and acquaintances as more important than those of older people is pervasive (see also Cadow, 1980).

One way in which younger people's needs are given priority over older people's is the provision of 'respite' care, either day or residential, for the benefit of relatives who are caring for older people. It is not disputed that those caring for older people who are severely disabled need breaks from this demanding work. Norman (1986) points out that it is ageist to assume that an old person's perceived needs should take precedence over all other considerations. The timing and type of care required, however, needs to be considered, bearing in mind the needs of both the client and the carer. Such an arrangement would be to their mutual benefit — many who care for older people refuse offers of respite care since they worry that the type of care offered will be detrimental to their relative's well-being. The authors found that movement of elderly clients from daytime attendance at a centre to short-stay Part III accommodation rarely involved any consideration of what effect this might have on the elderly client (Baldwin, 1986; Barrowclough and Fleming, 1986). Rehabilitative work with these clients at the day centre was severely interrupted when clients were temporarily removed from residential establishments to give breaks to carers.

This lack of regard for the rights of older people, particularly those who have a physical or mental handicap, may derive in part from the tendency to see age, or rather age-related disability, as having explanatory power. Thus, if a person who is suffering from dementia is removed temporarily from his or her own home into residential accommodation or to a Day

Centre, behaviours such as 'attempts to leave the establishment' or 'verbal abuse to staff' may well be construed not as indications of dissent with the placement but rather as 'symptoms' of the dementia. Goldiamond (1976) describes this approach as pathological: 'By describing apathy, depression or aggression as development stages in injury (or ageing), the staff is relieved of asking how their actions might have been causal'.

INFORMED CONSENT

Other authors have examined the ethical issues present in research with elderly people (e.g. Harris *et al.*, 1977). Much research concerns the elimination of age-related ailments and extending life. To this extent, it is 'anti-ageing' research but how this benefits elderly people is unknown, and therefore its goals require moral justification. Old people are more vulnerable to selection for research because of their unique physiological and psychological conditions, also because of their reduced freedom of action and competence. This vulnerability, which can lead to disproportionate selection for participation in research programmes, alerts us to the issue of consent, especially amongst institutionalized older people whose physical, mental, economic and social conditions all predispose them to exploitation. Effects of living in institutional settings (environmental and programme restraints, the fostering of dependence, demeaning treatment) all reduce an individual's ability to make competent and free choices to participate in research (Berkowitz, 1978). 'When persons are seen regularly to engage in activities which, were they stronger or in better circumstances, they would avoid, respect dictates that they will be protected against those forces that appear to compel their choices' (Reich, 1978).

Consent — whether to participate in research or therapeutic intervention — is a complex issue. It is commonly accepted that consent must always be qualified by the word 'informed'. This raises the question of whether an individual thoroughly understands the probabilities and/or complications connected with any procedures being advised. Does the person give assent, therefore, from an informed position? Consideration also needs to be given to the manner in which such information is conveyed, as this will influence the 'validity' of the consent obtained (i.e. does the person understand the information conveyed?). In institutions — and in families — is the individual's decision independent of pressure and is it made as a function of the older person's own needs rather than those of family members? This leads people to ask whether the Principle of Autonomy, noted earlier, should therefore take precedence over other principles. If it is decided that an individual is incapable of giving informed consent (e.g. because of severe cognitive impairment) how and by whom are decisions made on behalf of that person? This raises the issue of advocacy, which is explored further in Chapter One. One argument states that this is never justified and that there are grave moral risks in assuming 'guardianship' in this way. Reich (1978) suggests that a surrogate can only give consent in this way if he or she has exactly the same values as the individual in question and asserts that in the use of competence and guardianship, 'there is a crucial distinction only at an advanced age: the former have never had a set of personal values, while the latter have'.

Thus, the conflict between the desire to allow the individual freedom of choice (the Principle of Autonomy), and the desire to maximize his or her options to be able to continue to make decisions freely, is one dilemma commonly experienced in working with elderly people. This applies both inside and outside institutions, although decision-making on behalf of clients takes place more regularly within institutions and often in the absence of explicit guidelines.

In a discussion of the rights and risks which should be available to older people, Norman (1981) cites instances in which doctors have been able to overrule the decision of patients if the latter are thought to be 'not mature or lucid enough' to make such decisions. In this way the Principle of Autonomy is undermined by a premise of paternalism (the Principle of Beneficence, perhaps) that decisions are better made *for* someone who is older rather than by the person: in this case, with a sympathetic doctor, other professionals could be substituted in similar situations. (See also Gadow, 1980).

Goldiamond (1974, 1975) has addressed the issue of coercion in thera-peutic intervention and suggested that the functional analysis of coercive events can free them from being described simply in ethical terms and, furthermore, can make an intervention more amenable to 'counter-control' by the subject.

The idea that older people's wishes can be overruled is underlined by the 1948 National Assistance Act (although used infrequently) concerning the compulsory removal of older people from their homes into care, and the notion of 'rehabilitation'. Norman (1986) asks: 'Who benefits from the treatment? Who decides what is necessary? . . . Like other individuals, older people in residential homes should be able to refuse treatment and live with the consequences'. The contracts exchanged when a person enters residential care in East Sussex are offered as examples of possible ways to overcome these problems.

The overruling of old people's preferences by service agents is all the more questionable when evidence is presented that, frequently, service agents are negatively biased in their perceptions of older clients. Challis and Davies (1986) discuss the evidence for the unpopularity of social work with older clients, and the range of interventions considered tend to be narrow and undertaken with relatively low expectation of positive out-come. Kwiteck *et al.* (1986) demonstrated how American physical thera-pists were less 'aggressive' in their treatment of goal setting for old people than for a young person. These studies emphasize the need to consider possible conflicts of interest between the client and the service provider. The Kings Fund Centre document (1986a) in its discussion of services for dementia sufferers draws attention to such conflicts:

> The more intellectually impaired they (the older individual) become, the less likely they are to have an influence on their own existence. If people cannot/do not participate in the decisions which affect their lives, the conflicts of interest become a growing problem. Day in, day out, service providers interpret other people's needs in ways which reflect other priorities and constraints.

The document recommends advocacy as a partial solution. When people are unable to exert control over decisions affecting their lives, 'other advocacy' takes over — often that of professionals who are involved with the person. Their interests as professionals, however, may conflict with those of the older person. The document suggests that 'citizen advocates' can fulfil a valuable role by acting on behalf of elderly people to counteract the powerful role of professionals and institutions. Discussion includes the complexities of this task and potential problems which can arise.

INSTITUTIONAL LIVING

The key problems, which have already been discussed — decision-making and informed consent — are particularly salient in work in institutions, since such environments are strongly associated with the development of passivity and dependence; these factors are likely to result in difficulties in making decisions (Steinberg *et al.* 1986). Goffman (1961) was one of the earliest writers to highlight the problems for staff and inmates alike, including loss of individuality and general poverty of the social environment. Although only a small proportion of people over 65 in this country live in long-term residential care (RCP, 1988), this amounts to many people. Although there is a welcome move to people living in smaller units, research with other populations in residential care (e.g. Schroeder and Henes, 1978) has indicated that it is possible for institutional practices which have negative effects on clients, to develop in small and highly staffed settings. Townsend (1962) described the lack of activity among residents, and the lack of opportunity for participation in activity, as distinctive features in institutions caring for elderly people. More recently, Hughes and Wilkin (1980) in a review of the literature on quality of life in residential homes for elderly people, concluded that little had changed in 20 years, with residents sitting around the walls and lounges, neither communicating nor engaging in purposeful activities of any sort. In the USA, Baltes and colleagues (1980) have shown how dependent (rather than independent) behaviour of elderly residents in institutions is encouraged and maintained by staff. Burgio (1987) concludes that: '. . . the loss of adaptive functioning in many of the institutionalized elderly is not solely a result of biological decline but, to a large extent, a result of an environment that sets the occasion for and reinforces ineffective and dependent behaviour'.

The behaviour analyst who is asked to solve problems in such settings is likely to face difficulties. The ageing process is viewed by the behaviourist as an interaction between a biologically maturing individual and his or her immediate environment. Socially acceptable and independent-related behaviour is maintained throughout the ageing process only if the environment interacts with the individual by providing on-going support for this behaviour (Patterson and Jackson, 1980). Thus, if an older resident has socially unacceptable or excessively dependent behaviours, then the behaviour analyst will know that adaptive change will likely necessitate change in staff practices and increased prosthetics rather than in change within the resident. Given that the likely referring agent is the officer in charge of the institution, the problem for which help is requested is likely to be the reduction of some excess behaviour such as 'shouting' or 'aggression'.

It has been suggested that the applications of behaviour modification in institutions have been problematic as they have all too often been used as a means of enforcing traditional institutional values of, 'cleanliness, order, punctuality, deference and demeanour'. Given the evidence from a literature search which found that the client was rarely consulted in the choice of treatment goals and that the goals were institution-centred rather than for the benefit of the client, the ethical concerns find empirical support (see also Rebok and Hoyer, 1971). In the words of O'Donohue *et al.* (1986), 'The practice of using behaviour modification to enforce traditional institutional routine in nursing homes and geriatric wards was common'.

How should the behaviour therapist respond to the pressures to reduce or eliminate problem behaviours in such settings? The legitimacy of doing so, and the necessity of overriding the wishes of the 'problem' resident, often find expression in such statements as: 'we've got the rest of the residents to consider'. The authors sometimes would advocate the use of the constructional approach (e.g. Fleming *et al.* 1983) because the development of more adaptive behaviours will most often require changes in staff practices. Attempts at intervention, if worthwhile, very often require a fundamental restructuring of their context of application if they are to be successful. Less ambitious changes are possible if they do not conflict with the institution too greatly (Rebok and Hoyer, 1971).

APPROPRIATE GOALS FOR OLDER PEOPLE

Davies (1982) has made the point that 'those interested in behavioural work with the elderly adopt too narrow a perspective . . .', ignoring social psychological aspects and the ecological framework. If a behaviour analyst selects a goal for increase of independence of an older person in an institution where staff reinforce dependency, he or she may be frustrated by the outcome. Should independence be encouraged, particularly when the older person does not wish to engage in tasks? The guidelines which are used to assess, or at least to consider, needs with younger client groups may not be equally applicable to older people. For example, common to most assessment forms are questions about the adequacy of people's skills — domestic, personal, social etc. — and also their opportunities to participate in these activities. The assumption is that people 'need' a certain level of meaningful activity and social contact and that the loss of these functions from a person's repertoire is detrimental to their well-being. There is some theoretical and empirical support for these ideas from the behavioural literature, at least with younger people, and Skinner (1983) would argue that the laws of learning do not change with age. Does ageing involve a withdrawal from social activity by the older individual (Cumming and Henry, 1961)? Or is there no difference between old and young people in their need for social participation (Havinghurst, 1968)? Although there is some evidence (Abrams, 1980) that older people are not as socially active as younger age groups, Knapp's (1976) study of life satisfaction in older people and its relationship to social participation, did not provide evidence that this decrease in activity had a functional value (McFadyn, 1984).

Skinner (1983) argues that many changes in old age are due to changes in reinforcement contingencies. Thus, an elderly person who might be described as 'unmotivated' (to socialize, for example), would be described as not being sufficiently reinforced:

> In old age, behaviour is not so strongly reinforced. Biological ageing weakens reinforcing consequences. Behaviour is more and more likely to be followed by aches and pains and quick fatigue. Things tend to become 'not worth doing' in the sense that the aversive consequences exact too high a price. Positive reinforcers become less common and less powerful. Poor vision closes off the world of art, poor hearing the fidelitous music. Foods do not taste as good and erogenous tissues grow less sensitive. Social reinforcers are attenuated. Interests and tastes are shared with a smaller and smaller number of people.
>
> (Skinner, 1983)

Thus, ageing may reduce the availability of consequences in the person's environment which were critical reinforcers of behaviour, and inactivity can result. A much larger effort may therefore be needed to obtain these consequences. These points should be considered before one concludes that an old person 'just wants to sit' or is 'unmotivated'. The costs and benefits to an older individual of engaging in particular behaviour must be carefully evaluated if they are to make a real choice about changing their behaviour. Environmental modification in which known sources of reinforcement are readily available to the individual may be considered:

> What is needed is a prosthetic environment in which, in spite of reduced biological capacities, behaviour will be relatively free of aversive consequences and abundantly reinforced. New repertoires may well be needed as well as new sources of stimulation. . . . Our culture does not abundantly reinforce the behaviour of elderly people.
>
> (Skinner, 1983)

Accepting that the reasons for inactivity may be more to do with the environment than the person, if the older person consents to change, one is still left with the dilemma; 'is engagement in staff-directed activity of more "value" than private review of the past? Kushlick suggests using "engaged adaptive activity" as an index of quality of care but this still leaves open the criteria by which behaviours are to be judged adaptive . . . if, however, physical survival is used as a criterion of successful adaptation, aggressive self-centred behaviour may signify better adjustment' (Davies, 1982).

Independence is often seen as a goal and yet Goldiamond (1976) argues that we also need to accept dependency, since none of us — whatever our age or level of disability — is independent of our environment. To Goldiamond, the appropriate questions relate to whatever behavioural patterns, and under what conditions, elderly persons are dependent on the environment and in different ways from how they used to be (or how younger people are) dependent. And how can patterns of behaviour be developed or enhanced? If these patterns of behaviour are valued socially, then we should be doing our utmost to enable them to happen. In this way, the emphasis should be on the new conditions necessary for goals to be attained. 'Independence', as such, is not a useful way of describing goals for older people.

One dilemma with older people concerns their inactivity. Should attempts be made to overcome this and is 'activity' an appropriate goal of intervention? Goldiamond (1976) sees inactivity and apathy as a product of a person's environment and not a consequence of 'old age' with its assumed quality of choice.

Some of the activities in 'reality orientation' packages (e.g. Holden and Woods, 1982) which have been used in institutional settings for old people have been criticized on the grounds of being age and culture-inappropriate (Burton, 1982). It is suggested that some of these activities, such as spelling games and copying down information from a weatherboard, would be more appropriate for children than for older adults.

Burton (1982) has suggested that appropriate goals can be identified by examining the lifestyles of older people who are active and valued members of the community. This may lead to bias in favour of middle class older people and introduces the debate of how activities become 'valued' in the first place (see also de Beauvoir 1979). Burton returns to the theme of advocacy when suggesting that for more disabled older people, who will find the achievement of more valued goals too difficult, suggestions can be generated in co-operation with various Health and Social Service staff and volunteers, and perhaps the help of independent elderly people can be enlisted to review proposals.

CONCLUSIONS

The foregoing may represent a rather bleak picture of current practices in services for older people. Our purpose has been to draw attention to key problems which are likely to be of concern to all professionals who work with older clients and, particularly, to behaviour analysts. Central to these problems is a tendency to overlook the wishes of the older client and to give priority to other younger people whose preferences are given more value. A number of associated difficulties have been discussed, including: coercion in research and 'therapeutic' interventions, particularly in institutions, and the methods and pitfalls of assessing what are the appropriate goals for older people. Lack of education about such problems may lead the practitioner inadvertently to violate the rights of older people. Gilhooly (1986), in her discussion of the ethical issues arising from work with older people, comments on the lack of ethics teaching during the training of psychologists and other health care professionals.

Some recent behavioural literature has begun to inform practitioners of the need to assess their methods of work with older people and to recommend that client participation is always enlisted when interventions are made. Examples include the constructional approach (Goldiamond, 1974; 1976) and interventions such as goal planning. (Barrowclough and Fleming, 1986). Behavioural interventions should possess an inherent advantage to the client in the explicit statement of the intervention's goal and strategy for achieving them. In doing so, the ability of those receiving the intervention to exercise counter-control should be enhanced. The constructional approach, which increases rather than decreases the range of behaviours available to an individual, should also be encouraged and researched (Cullen *et al.*, 1981). Recent policy statements have suggested the development of advocacy for older people who may be unable to assert themselves fully. Although a complex issue, the employment of advocates within services for older people may help professionals to overcome some of the confusions and dilemmas referred to in the chapter and may lead to greater acknowledgement of the value of the older person.

REFERENCES

Abrams, M. (1980) *Beyond Three-score and Ten: A Second Report on a Survey of the Elderly*. Age Concern, Mitcham.

Baldwin., S. (1986) Systems in transition — the first 100 clients. Implication of developing specialist units for elderly people. *International Journal of Rehabilitation Research* **9** (2), 139–148.

Baltes, M. M., Burgess, R. L. and Stewart, R. B. (1980) Independence and dependence in self-care behaviour in nursing home residents: an operant-observational study. *International Journal of Behavioural Developments*, **3**, 489–500.

Barrowclough, C. and Fleming, I. (1986) Training direct care staff in goal planning with elderly people. *Behavioural Psychotherapy*, **14**, 192–209.

de Beauvoir, S. (1977) *Old Age*. Penguin, Harmondsworth.

Bender, M. P. (1986) The neglect of the elderly by British Psychologists. *Bulletin of the British Psychological Society*, **39**, 414–417.

Berkowitz, S. (1978). Informed consent. Research on the elderly. *The Gerontologist*, **18**, 237–243.

Burgio, L. D. (1987) Behavioural Staff Training and Management in Geriatric Long-term Care Facilities. In Wisocki, P. (ed.), *Clinical Behaviour Therapy for the Elderly*. Plenum Press, New York.

Burton, M. (1982). Reality orientation for the elderly: a critique. *Journal of Advanced Nursing*, **7**, 427–433.

Cadow, S (1980). Medicine, ethics and the elderly. *The Gerontologist*, **20**, 680–685.

Challis, D. and Davies, B. (1986) *Case Management in Community Care*. Gower Medical, London.

Cullen, C., Hattersley, J. and Tennant, L. (1981) Establishing behaviour: the constructional approach. In Davey, G. (ed.) *Applications of Conditioning Theory*. Methuen, London.

Cumming, E. and Henry, W. E. (1961) *Growing Old: The Process of Disengagement*. Basic Books, New York.

Davies, A. D. M. (1982) Research with the elderly people in long-term care: some social and organizational factors affecting psychological interventions. *Ageing and Society*, **2**, 285–297.

Denham, M. (1984) Ethics of research. *Nursing Mirror*, **158** (3), 36–38.

Estes, C. L. (1983). Austerity and ageing in the United States: 1980 and beyond. In Guillemard, A. M. (ed.) *Old Age and the Welfare State*. Sage Publications, London.

Fleming, I., Barrowclough, C. and Whitmore, R. (1983). The Constructional Approach to meeting the needs of elderly people. *Nursing Mirror*, **156** (23), 21–23.

Gilhooly, M. L. M. (1986). Ethical and legal issues in therapy with the elderly. In Hanley, I. and Gilhooly, M. (eds.) *Psychological Therapies with the Elderly*. Croom Helm, London.

Goffman, I. (1961) *Asylums: Essays on the Social Situations of Mental Patients and Other Inmates*. Doubleday, New York.

Goldberg, E. M. and Warburton, R. W. (1979) *Ends and Means in Social Work*. Allen and Unwin, London.

Goldiamond, I. (1974) Towards a constructional approach to social problems.

Ethical and constitutional issues raised by applied behaviour analysis. *Behaviourism*, **1**, 1–84.

Goldiamond, I. (1975) Alternative sets as a framework for behavioural formulations and research. *Behaviourism*, **3**, 49–86.

Goldiamond, I. (1976) Coping and adaptive behaviours of the disabled. In Albrecht, G. L. (ed.) *Socialisation in the Disability Process*. University of Pittsburgh Press, Pittsburgh.

Harris, S. L., Synder, B. D., Synder, R. L. and Magrow, B. (1977) Behaviour modification therapy with elderly demented patients: implementation and consideration. *Journal of Chronic Disability*, **30**, 129–134.

Havinghurst, I. G. (1968) Personality and patterns of ageing. *The Gerontologist*, **8**, 20–23.

Holden, U. P. and Woods, R. T. (1982) Reality orientation: Psychological approaches to the confused elderly. Churchill Livingstone, Edinburgh.

Hughes, R. B. and Wilkin, D. (1980). *Residential Care of the Elderly. A Review of the Literature*. Unpublished report, University of Manchester.

Kings Fund Centre (1986a) *Living Well into Old Age*. Project Paper No. 63. Kings Fund Centre, London.

Kings Fund Centre (1986b) *The mentally frail elderly: should we prescribe care?* Proceedings of a Conference held on March 25th, 1986. Kings Fund Centre, London.

Knapp, M. R. J. (1976) Predicting the dimensions of life satisfaction. *Journal of Gerontology*, **31**, 595–604.

Krasner, L. and Ullmann, L. P. (1973). *Behaviour Influence and Personality*. Pergamon, New York.

Kwiteck, S. D. B., Shaver, B. J., Blood, H. and Shepard, K. F. (1986) Age bias: physical therapists and older patients. *Journal of Gerontology*, **41**, 706–709.

McFadyn M. (1984) The measurement of engagement in the institutionalized elderly. In Hanley, I. and Hodge, J. (eds.) *Psychological Approaches to the Care of the Elderly*, Croom Helm, London.

Midwinter, E. (1986) Forced to be free. *International Journal of Geriatric Psychiatry*, **1**, 71–73.

Mosher-Ashley, P. M. (1987) Procedural and methodological parameters in behavioural-gerontological research: a review. *Int. J. Aging and Human Dev.*, **24** (3), 189–229.

Norman, A (1981). *Rights and Risk*. National Corporation for the Care of Old People, London.

Norman, A. (1986) *Aspects of Ageism: A Discussion Paper*. Centre for Policy on Ageing, London.

O'Donohue, W. T., Fisher, J. E. and Krasner, L. (1986) Behaviour therapy and The elderly: A conceptual and ethical analysis. *International Journal of Ageing and Human Development*, **23**, 1–15.

Patterson, R. L. and Jackson, G. M. (1980) Behaviour modification and the elderly. In Hersen, M., Miller, P. and Eisler, R. M. (eds.) *Progress In Behaviour Modification*. Academic Press, New York.

Patterson, R. L. (1982) *Overcoming deficits of ageing. A behavioural approach*. Plenum Press, New York.

Peterson, R. G., Knapp, T. J., Rosen, J. O. and Pither, B. F. (1977) The effects of furniture arrangement. *Behaviour Therapy*, **8**, 464–468.

Phillipson, C. and Walker, A. (1986) *Ageing and Social Policy: A Critical Assessment*. Gower Medical, London.

Powell-Lawton, M (1985) The elderly in context. *Environment and behaviour*, **17**, 501–519.

Rebok, G. W. and Hoyer, W. J. (1971) The functional context of elderly behaviour. *Gerontologist*, **17**, 27–32.

Reich, W. T. (1978) Ethical issues related to research involving elderly subjects. *The Gerontologist*, **18**, 326–337.

Royal College of Psychiatrists (1988) Long-stay beds for the elderly severely mentally ill. *Bulletin of the Royal College of Psychiatrists*, **12**, 250–2.

Schroeder, S. and Henes, C. (1978) Assessment of progress of institutionalized and deinstitutionalized retarded adults: A matched-control comparison. *Mental Retardation*, **16**, 147–148.

Skinner, B. F. (1983) Intellectual self-management in old age. *American Psychologist*, **38** (3), 239–44.

Slater, R. S. (1980) Residents' Rights of refusal. *Concorde*, **16**, 33–37.

Slivinske, L. R. and Fitch, V. L. (1987) The effect of control enhancing interventions on the well-being of elderly individuals living in retirement communities. *The Gerontologist*, **27**, 176–181.

Steinberg, A., Fitten, L. J. and Kachuck, N. (1986) Patient participation in treatment and decision-making in the nursing home: the issue of competence. *The Gerontologist*, **26**, 362–366.

Townsend, P. (1962) *The Last Refuge. A Survey of Residential Institutions and Homes for the ages in England and Wales*. Routledge, Kegan and Paul, London.

Walker, A. (1983) Social Policy and Elderly People — Great Britain. In Guillemard, A. M. (ed.) *Old Age and the Welfare State*, Sage Publications, London.

Zangwill, O. (1980) *Behaviour Modification: A report of a Joint Working Party to Formulate Ethical Guidelines for the Conduct of Programmes of behaviour Modification in the NHS*. HMSO, London.

Chapter Six

Working with people with a mental handicap

PHILIP DARBYSHIRE

EDITORS' INTRODUCTION

Recognition of the special needs of people with a mental handicap is relatively new. For centuries people with disparate disabilities were defined as similar to one another, although rarely treated as equal to the rest of humanity. The resulting myth of mental handicap has been a powerful stereotype: the heterogenity of people who are inherently different has often been overlooked. The recognition that people with different needs might require different services also was overlooked.

New, or more appropriate, services cannot, however, be built on the old foundations. The myths associated with mental handicap need 'deconstructing'. Part of the problem lies in the 'catch all' label of mental handicap: where people with only minor learning difficulties are included with others with major physical, emotional and intellectual handicaps. The assumption that all people with a mental handicap are handicapped in the same way, or to the same extent, needs to be challenged. The accompanying assumption that all people with mental handicaps have the same needs, and that they share none of the needs of the rest of humanity, also needs to be challenged.

In this chapter **Philip Darbyshire** traces some of the historical developments in the care of people with a mental handicap, emphasizing the feelings shown towards this group, some of the belief systems which underpin care practices, and the specific ethical issues which arise.

Working with people with a mental handicap

In recent years there has been a vast increase in interest in ethical issues relating to all aspects of health care. Mental handicap has been one area that, at times, has seemed like a mental adventure playground for philosophers, ethicists, doctors, nurses, and, increasingly, media commentators.

The issues that have tended to attract the most attention and comment have been the more dramatic 'life or death' dilemmas, such as those involving resuscitation or non-treatment of handicapped children, or sterilization of women or girls with a mental handicap.

While these dilemmas are important, they are not, unfortunately, issues in which nurses play a significant part. The concentration of attention on such headline-grabbing subjects also tends to detract attention from equally important ethical issues which care staff face in their daily contact with people with a mental handicap; indeed, care staff often find it difficult to recognize the ethical dilemmas which present themselves in the course of a day's work.

Some of these more 'every day' ethical concerns which affect all those who work with people with a mental handicap will be discussed, with ways in which these ethical problems may be approached.

WHAT'S IN A NAME?

The field of mental handicap has a history replete with some of the most colourfully abusive and derogatory description of people. Most workers in mental handicap are familiar with old terminology such as 'idiot', 'imbecile', 'moron', 'feeble-minded', 'moral defective', 'subnormal', 'retardate', 'mental defective', 'low-grade', and many others. In the present day it is all too easy to look back at these descriptions of people and wonder how they could possibly have been acceptable, even 50 years ago. This is a rather naive response, however, which fails to consider that these phrases were not simply descriptions but were clear indicators of the value of society at that time and an equally clear indication of how those societies viewed people with a mental handicap. Today's terminology of mental handicap speaks of 'people with a mental handicap', 'mentally handicapped people', 'special children', 'exceptional children', 'the cognitively disabled' and 'intellectual impairment'. Such a shift in language reflects a much wider shift in society's attitudes towards handicap and disability, but is this important for care staff? Does it really matter what we call people with a mental handicap?

In considering this question, a definite ethical problem is unanswered. Are there ethically correct or acceptable or desirable ways to describe people with a mental handicap and, if there are, what are they? Before considering this, it is useful to look at the whole purpose of 'labelling' a person or section of the population. It is clear that the labels of 'moron' or 'moral defective' served a purpose; that of clearly portraying the uselessness, undesirability and dangerousness of people with a mental handicap. Labelling can however be used to more positive purpose. Kopelman (1984) argues that labelling can have three positive benefits for people with a mental handicap:

Labelling may benefit the person where the label draws attention to the person's needs for particular help and therapeutic intervention. For example, a child who is diagnosed and labelled as having a visual defect may then benefit from opthalmic assistance and perhaps glasses. This benefit is not always self-evident and may be countered by the stigma associated with some diagnostic labels such as epilepsy (or, most recently and most dramatically, AIDS).

Labelling also may have benefits for society when a person with uncontrolled epilepsy may not be allowed to drive a car or fly an aircraft as this could endanger the lives of others. Again, the difficulty lies in balancing the person's rights to as 'normal' a lifestyle as is possible, with the rights of everyone else not to be endangered by the possible exercising of those rights. In this situation it is clearly important to be as confident as possible, that the 'danger' posed by the person is genuine and not merely the result of ignorance and prejudice.

Labelling can also be important for 'accuracy, or for integrity of observation' (Kopelman, 1984) where, for example, precise records need to be kept of epidemiological data regarding a rare clinical syndrome.

There can be no justification for the continued use of the most derogatory terminology but this seems to be a swipe at the flimsiest of straw men. Institutions, such as mental handicap hospitals, are notably slow to change the practices of past years and many nurses and other care staff in such hospitals will still encounter people who talk of 'low grades' (Hughes *et al.*, 1987) or the 'cot and chair' wards (Alaszewski, 1986), or devise their own abusive terminology for people with a mental handicap such as the 'cabbage patch kids', 'the vegetables' or 'the dopes' ward (*sic*).

Are there more positive ways to describe people with a mental handicap? As Kopelman (1984) argues, it is unlikely that there is such a thing as a truly value-free terminology of mental handicap; as the very act of defining handicap creates such values and obligations towards the person with a handicap. Most books and journal articles today seem to have adopted 'people with a mental handicap' as the most acceptable description as opposed to the previously more common 'mentally handicapped people'. The reason most frequently given for this preference is that the first phrase places more emphasis on the idea that people are *people* first and foremost and that their handicaps are almost a secondary consideration to this all important principle. There are, however, other ways to consider these terms. The phrase 'person with a mental handicap' is also unsatisfactory, however, for the reason that it seems to imply a dissociation between the person and his or her handicaps, as if the handicaps were almost tagged on to the person, instead of being an integral part of his or her life. In time, when nurses are being encouraged to adopt holistic (and wholistic) views of people, it seems regressive to suggest that their handicaps are not somehow a major part of their lives.

FEELINGS ABOUT PEOPLE WITH A MENTAL HANDICAP: RESPECT, TOLERANCE OR WORSE

In an avowedly human service, such as nursing or any other caring service serving people with a mental handicap, the quality of human contact between the care staff and people with a mental handicap is paramount. The crucial question is on what ethical principles can this human inter-action be based?

Most writers on ethics identify three fundamental moral principles which can be used to guide ethical behaviour and decision-making. These are **respect** for persons, **justice** and **beneficence**. While these principles can provide a good guide, they are not an infallible prescription for ethical behaviour and indeed they can often seem to be in opposition.

Respect for persons is a principle to which many care staff claim adher-ence. In nursing, the concept of treating patients as individuals has been encouraged for many years. Attempts to formalize this process through the unfortunately titled 'nursing process' and accompanying care plans have met with varying degrees of success. Similarly, in many mental handicap settings, care staff will be familiar with Individual Programme Plans (Jenkins, *et al.*, 1987). The concept of 'respect for persons' is more complex than it may first appear. For example, Downie (1985) asks: 'What is the formal object of the attitude of respect?', '. . . why are persons regarded as valuable?' and 'why then do we respect or value persons?' The extensive debate in philosophical circles as to what exactly makes a person (and who should therefore be considered as persons and who should not) is of relevance to this discussion but largely outwith the scope of this chapter.

The issue of personhood is as important for those caring for people with a mental handicap as it is as vitally important for those people in their care. Philosophers, such as Singer (1980), have been leading proponents of what might be called the 'criteria' or 'checklist' approach to personhood. Fletcher (1972; 1974) argues that 'any individual of the species homo-sapiens who falls below the IQ 40 mark in a standard Stanford-Binet test . . . is questionably a person; below the 20 mark, not a person'. Tooley (1985) uses a similar criteria approach, saying that to be considered as a person, one must '. . . be capable of action', 'possess self-consciousness' and 'rationality'.

There are many people with a mental handicap who could not fulfil these criteria. If you are working in a ward or unit with, for example, children with a mental handicap, are those children 'persons', 'fellow human beings' or something else? The 'something else' is synonymous with 'something less' — something less than people and something less than human. This question is relevant to any direct care setting, whether in a hospital or in the community. When staff begin to view the people in their care as somehow less than human, the groundwork is laid for every variety of neglect, sub-standard care and even physical abuse (Hewitt 1987; Martin 1984).

Kopelman (1984) argues that there are three main reasons why even persons with profound mental handicap are 'owed our respect as a fellow-being'. These are outlined as follows.

> First, they share a capacity to feel and their sentience should be respected. Second, as the discussion of labelling illustrated, how they are treated affects institutions; thus, it is in people's self-interests to see that they are treated respectfully. Third, beyond the minimal require-ments of sentience and self-interest, we share our communities and our homes with them; we respect the commitment, benevolent concern of affection that holds families together.

This is surely a more satisfactory way for care staff to view the personhood of people with a mental handicap, not as a set of rather arbitrary and intelligence-referenced criteria but as social beings who do not live in isolation and whose lives touch others; they are, in turn, affected by the attentions of those who care for them.

PATERNALISM: LOOKING FORWARD OR LOOKING AFTER?

Paternalistic control has been a cornerstone of the care of people with a mental handicap for many years. It had been widely accepted that, left to their own devices, people with mental handicap would be unable to ensure and safeguard their own health and welfare. For this reason, people with a mental handicap had to be 'looked after' and protected from themselves. Such protection ensured they were denied almost any measure of personal autonomy and control over their own lives. It is perhaps too easy to blame such a situation on care staff who may be accused of being too domineering and authoritative. This is to ignore the whole ethos of nursing in custodial care, whereby the person with a mental handicap was seen as largely incapable of exercizing any degree of autonomy or choice. Indeed, if such choices were encouraged, the smooth running of the institution would undoubtedly suffer.

Sadly for nurses and nursing, it was often assumed that the role of the nurse in caring for people with a mental handicap was to 'do everything that you can for them'. People with a mental handicap were viewed as children or babies who were largely incapable of exerting any control over their own lives and who constantly had to be observed, supervized and restricted 'for their own good'. Yet such views of nursing are a travesty of the true nature of nursing care. The concept of a style of nursing which emphasizes the nurse's central role in helping people to achieve greater autonomy and control over their own lives is not new. In 1969 the doyen of nurses, Virginia Henderson was writing that:

> The unique function of the nurse is to assist the individual, sick or well, in the performance of those activities contributing to health or its recovery or to a peaceful death, that he or she would perform unaided had he the strength, will or knowledge, and to do this in such a way as to help him achieve independence as rapidly as possible. (described in Fulton, 1987).

With its emphasis on the individual and on the importance of that person's independence, Henderson emphasized the importance of increasing autonomy as a prime nursing function.

It would be simplistic, however, to assume that paternalism is invariably bad and that autonomy is always to be preferred. In ethical issues, sound principles often come into conflict. For example, if a person with a mental handicap repeatedly ran on to a busy road, it would be absurd to suggest that the chosen desire to take this action should be allowed as this represents granting autonomy. Allowing the person to choose such a course of action is in conflict with principle of 'beneficence and duty to care' and the ensuring that harm is not done. Examples of this conflict between paternalism and autonomy are common in all care contexts. Should people with a mental handicap be allowed to choose where they should live and with whom? Should they be allowed to choose their own sexual and marital partners? Should they be allowed to enter into commercial and legal contacts? Or will these decisions be made by others, either parents or members of 'multi-disciplinary teams'?

Care staff should also address this problem when the capacity of persons with a mental handicap for autonomy is clearly and markedly diminished (as in the case of children with profound mental handicap for example). How do your communicate, verbally or by gesture? What do you do if a person with a mental handicap seems to want to sit in a chair rocking and making stereotyped movements with her hands all day? Do young children have any autonomy at all, or should they always be expected to conform to adult expectations?

There are of course no rule books or procedure manuals which can tell care staff when to 'allow' autonomy or when paternalistic intervention is the best course of action. Within the spirit of enlightened care of people with a mental handicap, wherever possible (and this includes many more situations than have been previously imagined) autonomy should be allowed and encouraged. As Boggs (1986) argues: 'Basic to the problem is an understanding that, in order to achieve competence, a person (child or adult) with mental retardation must know that he or she has choices, and that what he or she decides will make a difference'.

Care staff can encourage people with mental handicap to make choices in many ways. Mealtimes are a useful example of an area of direct care where choice could be further encouraged and where lack of choice can contribute towards mealtimes becoming mere 'refuelling stops' (Alaszewski, 1986). Are people allowed to choose what they would like to eat at mealtimes or do staff make up the menus without consulting them? Are people's food preferences catered for and their dislike of particular foods respected? Are people allowed to try to feed themselves, regardless of how messy or time-consuming this may be? The question of real choice is central to the idea of encouraging autonomy and independence, and can be applied to every aspect of the lives of people with a mental handicap; including work, leisure activities and social relationships.

The justification for paternalism is that it seeks to do what is best for the person. It is not by its very nature a form of neglect or mistreatment but, in the lives of people with a mental handicap, it can be yet another mechanism to prevent their living as normal a life as is possible (Khan, 1985). This life may include making mistakes and bad decisions but these are nonetheless decisions and, as such, have a value despite their undesired outcomes. It is not only non-handicapped people who should be allowed to learn from their mistakes.

PEOPLE WITH A MENTAL HANDICAP: MEANS OR ENDS?

There is a fundamental moral principle related to the concept of 'respect for persons' which states that people should be seen as ends in themselves and not merely as means to an end. This principle is important when considering various aspects of care and treatment. But what does it mean to treat someone as an 'end' or as a 'means'? This idea incorporates many aspects of our own personal beliefs and values, and those about the care setting where the person with a mental handicap may live. To treat a person with a mental handicap as an 'end' requires recognition that he or she is a unique individual to whom we have a duty of care. This also requires recognition of that person's individualism and also the autonomy and moral rights which he or she possesses (Hoffmaster, 1982). (See also Example 1 on page 96).

Examples of people with a mental handicap treated simply as 'ends' are all too commonly seen in care settings where the institution's 'needs' are deemed to be more important than the people who live there. Recognizing and fostering the growth and development of a person with a mental handicap as an individual is so important to the idea of treating people as 'ends', that in any care setting where people with a mental handicap are merely contained or treated in batches, or as homogenous groups, treating people as means to an end will be the norm. The end in question is usually a quieter life for care staff through a diminution of work, nuisance or bother, or the person's compliance with the rules and regulations of the institution.

Aspin (1982) argues forcibly for the principle of treating people as ends in themselves:

> We may reasonably ask whether we are justified in employing any techniques in the education of handicapped children that involves regarding them as in some respects less than persons or diminishing respects for their rights. We do this — we violate what Kant regarded as the prime principle of morality: that of not treating persons as means but only always as ends — whenever we treat children as inert lumps of organic matter whose acceptable or non-acceptable behaviour tendencies we discuss in their presence; when we fail to consider that the regime we prescribe for them might involve pain or distress; whenever we use means of treating them which amount to manipulation of them as things and do not solicit the conscious acts of voluntary engagement and assent of which the child might be minimally capable.

Encouragement of respect for a person's individuality, autonomy and personhood is, however, not always unproblematic. Deciding who should be involved in decisions about the person's care and treatment can be difficult. Clearly, the above principles demand that the person is closely involved in any such decisions. The trend in recent years of people demanding to be allowed to speak for themselves on matters concerning their lives is heartening (Williams and Schoultz, 1982). What is to be done, however, when the person's degree of handicap is so severe that 'real involvement' is not possible? This raises the problem of who is to speak for the best interests of the person with a mental handicap. Is it to be the parents? Is it to be medical staff who can claim that they have an ultimate legal responsibility? Is it to be nursing staff who are increasingly claiming to be 'the patient's advocate'? Is it to be a group of people — some form of multidisciplinary team who may or may not agree with a treatment decision? Or is it to be someone from an 'outside' organization such as 'Advocacy Alliance'?

There are problems with each of these possibilities, however. Encouraging individuals themselves to decide may be desirable, when their decisions are deemed acceptable. As Yule and Carr (1987) note, however:

> If we are to respect that individuality of a person with a mental handicap, shouldn't we allow him to express his likes and dislikes? Given that he cannot do so conventionally with spoken language, shouldn't we tolerate his hitting other residents? Apart from begging the question about the functional meaning of hitting, this form of argument ignores

two other important elements. First, other people also have rights: parents, siblings, other clients and staff have the right not to be assaulted. In any case, if a client is regularly aggressive, he will soon lose out socially and educationally. Second, on normalisation principles, clients should not be encouraged in behaviours that will stigmatise them in the community.

Professionals also have been criticized for almost automatically claiming this right to speak for the person with a mental handicap. Rothman (1982) argues that the track record of doctors and nurses in the residential care of people with a mental handicap has been so poor that they can scarcely claim this right: 'Who speaks for the retarded? The professionals? I'm sorry, I find that unconvincing. You don't have, from my perspective, a good deal of credit to go on'.

Nurses often claim to be patient's advocates, but against whom are they protecting the patient's interests? If it is the actions of other professionals, the nurse will find this extremely difficult, as shown by recent highly publicized cases of psychiatric nurses who refused to follow the doctor's instructions. Nurses' concepts of what were in the patient's best interests was clearly in conflict with those of medical staff and health authorities; indeed, the idea of the 'nurse as advocate' received short shrift. Nurses may also find that protecting patients' interests may sometimes involve protecting patients from actual physical abuse (Beardshaw, 1981).

Protection from psychological and emotional abuse can be even more difficult. Morgan (1987), in describing her experiences as a student nurse tells of the conflict that she experienced when she was a witness to patient abuse:

> I had always suppressed my guilt and the internal conflict I felt when I followed instructions of doubtful propriety. Continual rationalisation meant that I never challenged what I was being told to do; after all, I was new to the system; I needed a good report. I knew that reporting the incident would result in serious consequences. When it came to the crunch, although I had reported what I had seen, I was unable to name the member of staff concerned. As a result, in some ways I felt I had let the resident involved down as he was unable to speak and defend his own interests.

While this is a very realistic account of the mixed feelings that staff (especially junior or inexperienced staff) may have when they feel that mistreatment is occurring, the correct and ethically defensible course of action is very clear. 'But, at another level, staff are confronted with a frighteningly simple proposition — if they observe cruelty or neglect, severe or mild, it is their moral and professional duty to try to do everything in their power to see that it is stopped' (*Nursing Times*, 1983). This is an inescapable aspect of professional accountability.

THE ETHICAL BASIS OF INTERVENTIONS AND TREATMENT

In a busy ward or unit where people with a mental handicap live, it is too easy for staff to be so caught up in the momentum of 'getting the work done' that the philosophy of care which underpins the unit's function (and the considerations which should inform the work of the unit) are often forgotten. As Greenfield (1982) noted:

> In the terms of the day-to-day reality of living with the problem, it's a lot different. You don't have time to think of what's right, what is ethically right. You don't have time to think of the morality of something. You don't have time to think about all of these things because you're living in a crisis situation . . . How do you get this child not to destroy property? How do you get this child to eat food, to eat a balanced diet? When you have a child who's that way, it's very hard to see the overall. I guess one has to see it but one just doesn't.

Yet nurses and other care staff can pay a very heavy price for neglecting to discuss, describe and develop the theoretical and ethical bases for their work with people with a mental handicap. This price is often paid in the institutional currency of loss of idealism, professional depression, and an increasing hardness and cynicism towards their work and people with a mental handicap (Firth *et al.*, 1987).

Such a questioning process is not easy, for it raises many difficult questions which are not easily answered. Who is the subject of our treatment and intervention? Is it to be the person with a mental handicap only, or are we to adopt the notion that somehow a 'handicapped child' equals a 'handicapped family' and begin to involve parents and other relatives? Who is going to decide what form our treatments and interventions will take: professionals, parents, the person themselves, or a combination of everyone? Are all of these opinions about treatment to carry equal weight, or will one person's opinions override the others? How will we decide what areas of the person's life require our intervention? And how will we decide that it is time to end intervention and treatment? Is 'maximum potential' ever realized? (see Example 2 on page 97). It is not possible to discuss all of these questions but one aspect of this underlying philosophy, which many nurses and care staff claim to support and use in their work with people with a mental handicap, is the concept of normalization.

Normalization has been variously defined as helping mentally handicapped people to enjoy '. . . patterns and conditions of everyday life which are as close as possible to the norms and patterns of the mainstream of society' (Nirje, 1970), and, '. . . the utilisation of means which are as culturally normative as possible' (Wolfensberger, 1972). This involves use of services and facilities which are not segregated but which are used by a 'normal' or non-handicapped population. Although few people could disagree, even in seemingly uncontentious issues, there are ethical questions for staff.

Hoffmaster (1982) raises two possible objections to normalization. He has questioned whether the principle is '. . . to be understood as an end or a means'. If it is seen as an end, then the problems relate to whether the 'end' is ethically justifiable, especially if this end is interpreted as being that we should be trying to make the person with a mental handicap 'normal'. Hauerwas (1977) argues that:

> The great temptation in caring for the retarded, as for any child [*sic*], is to make them conform to what we think they should want to be — namely, that they should wish to be 'normal' . . . But, as an ideology, [normalization] tends to suggest that our aim is to make no clear idea of what it means to be 'normal'. Thus, in the name of 'normalcy', we stand the risk of making the retarded conform to convention because they lack the power to resist.

Similar problems exist with the concept of encouraging behaviours and experiences which are 'culturally normative'. Again, the aim is laudable: that the stigma and sense of difference, which is so pervasive in mental handicap, be reduced by encouraging a reduction in this cultural difference between handicapped and non-handicapped members of society. However, 'culturally normative' is not a value-neutral term and tends to suggest that our society is composed of one unified culture about which everyone agrees. As this is clearly not the case, we must decide into which culture we are attempting to help the person fit.

Another problem is that what is 'culturally normative' may not be desirable. Misuse of alcohol and drugs may be culturally normative for more young people but we would be loathe to encourage this in adolescents with a mental handicap. Other attempts to deal with this problem (by replacing the idea of 'normative' by the idea of 'valued') merely confronts us with similar difficulties in deciding which skills, characteristics and attributes are to be valued.

This is well illustrated in the well-known story of Jean Itard and his 'saving' of the so-called 'Wild Boy of Averyon' who had been living among wild animals in the woods. In Itard's world, the boy was seen as a savage incapable of functioning in the 'real' world. But what would have happened had Itard been hopelessly lost in the woods without food or shelter when he met his wild boy? Whose skills and abilities would have been most valuable in this world?

The purpose of this discussion is not to attempt to discredit the concept of normalization but to demonstrate that nurses and other caregivers are working with very complex theoretical and practical issues. These are not vague abstractions of interest only to academics, but have real and important ethical moral dimensions for practising caregivers.

CONCLUSIONS AND SUGGESTIONS

One of the difficulties for nurses and other caregivers which has already been mentioned is their ability to see that a problem, questions or idea may be an ethical dilemma. It is easy to recognize major moral controversies. However, often during a normal working day equally important (for the people concerned) ethical decisions are taken, albeit less consciously or deliberately. Nurses and other care staff should make deliberate and systematic attempts to identify the ethical concerns which they face daily and to encourage informed discussion of these issues.

While it is not possible to prescribe a 'correct' ethical response to every situation which care staff may encounter, some guidelines may be useful. Ethical principles, which stress the consequences of our actions, emphasize the importance of beneficence and 'normaleficence'; doing good, not harm, to others; while other principles emphasize the importance of justice and treating people fairly, respecting persons' autonomy and honesty and truthfulness in dealing with others. But, while such general principles are valuable, there are other principles which have been developed, specifically in relation to the care of people with a mental handicap.

Raine (1982) lists five 'moral axioms' against which she suggests can be measured 'the appropriateness of any treatment mode for handicapped people'. These are:

1. . . . any treatment mode employed should approximate to the greatest extent possible, those patterns and conditions of life which are the norms and patterns of the mainstream of society . . .
2. . . . the extent to which it (the treatment mode) inherently provides a humane environment . . .
3. . . . any treatment mode which is employed for use with mentally retarded people must be oriented to the maximization of their development potentials . . .
4. . . . each person coming under our care has a right to expert treatment that is professionally sound and competently administered . . .
5. . . . each handicapped person receive treatment which affirms his/her individuality.

Similar principles form the basis of the editorial policy of the journal *Community Living*, and although these are not claimed to be ethical principles they serve this function extremely well. They are (*Community Living*, 1987):

Increasing Choices — giving both people who use the service, and those who run them, a wider range of options in ways of living, working and playing;

Increasing individualization and privacy — making sure the services reflect respect for the uniqueness of each person;

Extending integration — working out ways of enabling consumers to mix with people who are not handicapped;

Improving participation — increasingly ensuring that consumers have a greater role in the running and management of the services they use;

Better relationships — moving towards treating consumers as colleagues.

Working towards the realization of such principles will not be easy. Ignoring the value of such principles may make 'helping' people with a mental handicap considerably harder in the long-term.

EXAMPLES

Example 1

'The Valley Hospital' had a programme of 'socialization' whereby residents were often taken into the nearby town to use public transport, visit the cinema, go for a meal, etc.. Staff Nurse Smith expressed his disagreement with the fact that only the 'good' and most capable residents seemed to be taken on these outings. He argued that residents with severe mental handicap and even those with 'behaviour problems' should be allowed the same right to use the facilities of the community.

Charge Nurse Jones was unhappy about this as he felt that the public acceptance of people with a mental handicap would not be best served by what he considered to be the 'shock tactics' of Staff Nurse Smith. He also suggested that Staff Nurse Smith was trying to use people with a mental handicap to implement his own personal philosophy of normalization and socialization.

Staff Nurse Smith rejected this, saying that if the public could not accept *all* people with a mental handicap, regardless of their handicaps, then that was their problem and was no reason to deprive certain residents of the opportunity of going on the outings.

Discussion points

What ethical principles, if any, underpin the positions taken by Staff Nurse Smith and Charge Nurse Jones? Is either Staff Nurse Smith or Charge Nurse Jones viewing people with a mental handicap as ends or as means?

If they are, what effect does this view have on their understanding of the situation?

What other ethical issues are raised in this situation?

Example 2

James is a 40 year old man with a severe mental handicap and who has lived in 'The Valley Hospital' since he was a young child. He will spend most of the day sitting in a chair in the ward making 'sterotyped' movements with his hands and flicking a small piece of wood or pencil between his fingers.

Staff believe that this is not an appropriate way for James to spend his day and, over several years, they have tried various treatment programmes and strategies to try to minimize James' mannerisms and to involve him in 'more valued' activities. These attempts, however, have been unsuccessful. During these, James had become extremely anxious, distressed and even violent; on one occasion even requiring to have an injection of a major tranquillizing drug.

At a case conference, at which another programme was suggested for James, Staff Nurse Black suggested that it was perhaps time to stop 'trying to interfere so much in James' life' by trying to change his lifestyle in ways that involved making him do things that he obviously did not want to do and which caused him such distress and unhappiness. Staff Nurse Black argued that James was expressing preference, in his own way, for the activities that he enjoyed and that staff should respect his wishes as they surely would if James were a non-handicapped person.

Staff Nurse Black's colleagues were rather taken aback at this and Miss White, a trainee clinical psychologist, was critical of Staff Nurse Black for being 'defeatist and pessimistic' and for suggesting in effect that nothing could be done for people like James.

Discussion points

How should people decide whether the behaviour of residents such as James', is acceptable or unacceptable?

Should the professionals always decide? What part is to be played in these decisions by the residents themselves?

Staff Nurse Black claimed that James' treatment programmes were causing him unacceptable distress and unhappiness. How can we balance any possible short-term resistance or unhappiness with the possibility that there may be long-term advantages for the person?

Is a point ever reached when 'enough is enough' regarding intervention and treatment programmes? If so, how is this point to be decided, and by whom?

Is it possible to reconcile Staff Nurse Black's position with nursing's general commitment to maximize independence and 'potential'?

REFERENCES

Alaszewski, A. (1986) *Institutional Care and the Mentally Handicapped: The Mental Handicap Hospital*. Croom Helm, London.

Aspin, D. N. (1982) Towards a concept of human being as a basis for a philosophy of special education. *Educational Review*, **34**(2), 113–123.

Beardshaw, V. (1981) *Conscientious Objectors at Work: Mental Hospital Nurses — A Case Study*. Social Audit, London.

Boggs, E. M. (1986) Ethics in the middle of life: An introductory overview. In Dokecki, P. R. and Zaner, R. M. (eds.) *Ethics of Dealing with Persons with Severe Handicaps: Towards a Research Agenda*. Paul H. Brookes, Baltimore.

Community Living Journal (1987) Statement of editorial policy. *Community Living*, **1**(2), 3.

Downie, R. S. (1985) Ambivalence of attitude to the mentally retarded. In Laura, R. S. and Ashman, A. F. (eds.) *Moral Issues in Mental Retardation*. Croom Helm, Beckenham.

Firth, H., McKeown, P., McIntee, J. and Britton, P. (1987) Professional depression, 'burnout' and personality in longstay nursing. *International Journal of Nursing Studies*, **24**(23), 227–237.

Fletcher, J. (1972) *Indicators of Humanhood: A Tentative Profile of Man*. Hastings Centre Report, **2**(1), 1–4.

Fletcher, J. (1974) *Four Indicators of Humanhood — The Enquiry Matures*. Hastings Centre Report, **4**(1), 4–7.

Fulton, J. S. (1987) Virginia Henderson: Theorist, prophet, poet. *Advances in Nursing Science*, **10**(1), 1–9.

Greenfield, J. (1982) Parents' forum. In Hauerwas, S. (ed.) *Responsibility for Devalued Persons: Ethical Interactions between Society, the Family and the Retarded*. C. C. Thomas, Springfield, Illinois.

Hauerwas, S. (1977) Having and learning how to care for retarded children: Some reflections. In Reiser, S. (ed.) *Ethics in Medicine*. MIT Press, Cambridge.

Henderson, V. (1969) *Basic Principles of Nursing Care*. International Council of Nurses, Basel.

Hewitt, S. E. (1987) The abuse of deinstitutionalized persons with mental handicaps. *Disability, Handicap and Society*, **2**(2), 127–135.

Hoffmaster, B. (1982) Caring for retarded persons: Ethical ideals and practical choices. In Hauerwas, S. (ed.) *Responsibility for Devalued Persons: Ethical Interactions between Society, the Family and the Retarded*. C. C. Thomas, Springfield, Illinois.

Hughes, D., May, D. and Harding, S. (1987) Growing up on Ward Twenty: the everyday life of teenagers in a mental handicap hospital. *Sociology of Health and Illness*, **9**(4), 378–409.

Jenkins, J., Felce, D., Mansell, J., de Kock, U. and Toogood, S. (1987) Organizing a residential service. In Yule, W. and Carr, J. (eds) *Behaviour modification for people with mental handicaps*. Croom Helm, Beckenham.

Khan, R. F. (1985) Mental retardation and paternalistic control. In Laura, R. S.

and Ashman, A. F. (eds.) *Moral Issues in Mental Retardation*. Croom Helm, Beckenham.

Kopelman, L. (1984) Respect and the retarded: issues of valuing and labelling. In Kopelman, L. and Moskop, J. C. (eds.) *Ethics and Mental Retardation*. Reidel/ Kluwer, Dordrecht.

Lane, H. (1977) *The Wild Boy of Averyon*, George Allen & Unwin, London.

Martin, J. P. (1984) *Hospitals in Trouble*. Basil Blackwell, Oxford.

Morgan, K. (1987) Through my eyes — one nursing student's view. In Parrish, A. (ed.) *Mental Handicap*. Macmillan, Basingstoke.

Nirje, B. (1970) The normalization principle — implications and comments. *British Journal of Mental Subnormality*, **16**(2), 62–70.

Nursing Times (1983) Editorial. **79**(30), July 27, 15.

O'Brien, J. and Tyne, A. (1981) *The principle of normalization: a foundation for effective services*. Campaign for Mentally Handicapped People, London.

Raine, B. (1982) The Limitations of Public Policy: Ethical dilemmas surrounding society's commitment to its mentally retarded members, in *Responsibility of Devalued Persons: Ethical interactions between society, the family and the retarded* (ed. S. Hauerwas), C. C. Thomas, Springfield, Illinois.

Rothman, D. J. (1982) Who speaks for the retarded? The rights and needs of devalued persons. In Hauerwas, S. (ed.) *Responsibility for Devalued Persons: Ethical Interactions between Society, the Family and the Retarded*. C. C. Thomas, Springfield, Illinois.

Singer, P. (1980) *Practical Ethics*. Cambridge University Press, Cambridge.

Tooley, M. (1985) *Abortion and Infanticide*. Oxford University Press, Oxford.

Williams, P. and Schoultz, B. (1982) *We can Speak for Ourselves*. Souvenir Press, London.

Wolfensberger, W. (1972) *The Principle of Normalization in Human Services*. National Institute for Mental Retardation, Toronto.

Yule, W. and Carr, J. (1987) *Behaviour Modification for People with Mental Handicaps*. Croom Helm, Beckenham.

Part Three

Chapter Seven

Autonomy and mental health

JAQUELINE ATKINSON

EDITORS' INTRODUCTION

Although the individuality of people is clear, independence is a more relative concept. Ideas about autonomy are inherently philosophical, if not even cultural. People are assumed to be self-determining, self-governing individuals. People reason, people choose: these functions set us apart from other animals. Traditionally, this concept has been challenged when applied to people with intellectual impairments or other 'mental' disabilities such as the major mental 'illnesses'. If the person's reasoning process is impaired, for whatever reason, is autonomy relinquished?

In this chapter **Jaqueline Atkinson** discusses the traditional concepts of autonomy and self-determination, and the development of ideas like 'paternalism' which were deemed appropriate for people who were considered not autonomous in some way. Is it feasible to describe all people as autonomous? What are the practical, as well as ethical problems of restricting the person's autonomy, or in allowing everyone the right to self-determination?

Autonomy and mental health

Morality has many dimensions including, possibly, a spiritual one, but as Downie and Calman (1987) point out: 'Whatever else morality may be, it is at least a set of principles which help us to live together in society more harmoniously and co-operatively than we could without it.' Thus, amongst other things, morality is a social device, and moral principles can be achieved by consensus. The many varied and detailed rules which govern our interaction with others derive from four basic principles of consensus morality: non-malfeasance, beneficence, justice and utility. Such principles imply an 'ought', that is, 'people ought to behave in certain ways' — out of a desire not to harm others, or to be of positive help to others, or to treat others fairly and equally or, lastly, to ensure the best possible outcome for the majority. Behaviour is thus seen to be, or 'ought to be' governed by principles other than simply self-interest. Where does the ethical authority for such moral principles come from?

These principles rest on the underlying belief in the autonomous person. Having respect for such an autonomous person, whether self or other, can be seen as the overriding ethical principle. This is set out by Kant. He says 'by mere analysis of the concepts of morality we can quite well show that the above principle of autonomy is the sole principle of ethics. Analysis finds that the principle of morality must be a categorical imperative, and that this in turn commands nothing more nor less than precisely this autonomy (trans. Paton, 1969).

This chapter considers autonomy in relation to the mental health of individuals, and how mental health problems can pose a number of dilemmas for society upholding the principle of respect for the autonomous person.

To be an autonomous person means to be able to choose for oneself, and can be seen to operate through two distinct areas, self-determination and self-government.

SELF-DETERMINATION

Self-determination involves individuals being able to formulate and carry out their own plans, desires, wishes and policies, thereby determining the course of their own life. It is usually accepted that this involves both the mental and physical capacity to make choices and then carry them out. A society which values autonomy will seek to maximize such choice. In contrast, life within a totalitarian regime is not necessarily painful. Such a regime can provide for the physical and material comfort of its members. People living under such a regime may even be happy and contented. This is not the point. Rather, the objections raised to such a society come from the centralized control over people's lives that the regime exerts. The assumption is that it is more important for humankind to exert free will, than it is to be contented. It is probably not possible to prove that well-fed, physically healthy, materially satisfied, contented people living as automata have lost their distinctive humanity, but it is a firmly held belief amongst those who oppose totalitarianism and support liberal democracy.

In any society the individual does not have full autonomy; political and social restraints are exercized to restrict choice. Thus not everyone has the same access to the health services, through both unequal provision of services and educational disadvantage or social custom which does not allow the person to make use of the services provided (Townsend and Davidson, 1982). Within this limitation we can describe conditions which are necessary to develop and practice an individual's capacity for autonomy. This involves having choices over lifestyle, religious and philosophical beliefs and practices, political beliefs and organization, choices over work, housing, travel and migration, education and relationships. It also involves having choices about one's physical and mental health. The organization of society, whether politically or through a cultural value system, can either restrict the range of images a person may have of themselves or impose certain images or norms of behaviour. This will be discussed further in the section on prescriptions for mental health.

Autonomy is only genuine when there is equal access to resources and we know that unequal access can affect mental health (Newton, 1988). Nevertheless, one can act with autonomy in as far as a given set of restricted circumstances allows. It is generally accepted that individuals have an over-riding interest in their own autonomy. This is not always the case, and a desire for autonomy and for happiness (or absence from pain) may conflict. Whilst classical utilitarianism may be seen to propose that the 'general good' or 'the general happiness' should prevail, Mill's (1859) defence of liberty is based on the principle that autonomy is the most valued aspect of Man, a view reiterated in his treatise on utilitarianism:

> Of two pleasures, if there be one to which all or almost all who have experience of both give a decided preference, irrespective of any feeling of moral obligation to prefer it, that is the more desirable pleasure. If one of the two is, by those who are competently acquainted with both, placed so far above the other that they prefer it, even though knowing it to be attended with a greater amount of discontent, and would not resign it for any quantity of the other pleasure which their nature is capable of, we are justified in ascribing to the preferred enjoyment a superiority in quality, so far outweighing quantity as to render it, in comparison, of small account.
>
> (Mill, 1861)

Mill sums up his argument in the memorable statement: 'It is better to be a human being dissatisfied than a pig satisfied; better to be Socrates dissatisfied than a fool satisfied.'

Although most restrictions on autonomy are believed to be through malfeasance, restrictions also occur through benevolence. Thus society or an individual might seek to restrain a person's freedom to formulate and carry out his or her own plans 'in that person's best interest'. This is the argument frequently used to impose 'treatment' on 'patients' whether they want it or not and will be discussed in greater detail in the section on paternalism and its application in the section on mental health problems.

SELF-GOVERNMENT

As well as self-determination, autonomy also requires that individuals are able to govern their own lives by rules and values. Being an autonomous person does not, therefore, eliminate the possibility that one's desires may be in conflict with values and rules by which one may want to prescribe both one's own behaviour and the behaviour of others. Indeed, for Kant, the mature person is able to place rules, governing others as well as self, above his or her own desires. 'Autonomy of the will' is the core of a 'rational being' as Kant described. Through rational choice, the highest elements of human nature are expressed at the expense of individual desires. He states 'the principle of autonomy is:' 'Never to choose except in such a way that in the same volition the maximums of your choice are also present as universal law'. This 'practical rule' is defined as 'an imperative — that is, that the will of every rational being is necessarily bound to the rule as a condition'. Kant's view of human nature is to separate the rational from the emotional, and to place greater value on the rational part.

Other views of human nature would not defend this dichotomy, and in this chapter the person will be considered as a unified whole: 'The autonomous person in his (*sic*) self-determination, self-governing and emotional reactions is a unity . . . the morally appropriate treatment of an autonomous person ought to be determined by awareness of this unified human nature' (Downie and Calman, 1987).

Autonomy is not the only principle of intrinsic value and although mental state utilitarianism (that is, to produce the greatest amount of pleasure over pain) may be compelling, there are times when autonomy conflicts with pleasure or other principles. Common examples are where one person's autonomy curtails that of another (i.e. would harm another person) or where short-term autonomy damages the long-term autonomy of the person. Using the example of suicide, short-term autonomy — the right to kill one's self — diminishes long-term autonomy: a corpse has no autonomy. On a less final note, it might be argued that using heroin to give pleasure is an autonomous choice the person has a right to make. It is, however, only a short-term autonomous choice, as in the long-term addicts have no choice about their dependence on the substance. If someone with an addiction to heroin genuinely wants to be free of this addiction, he or she may find long-term autonomy severely compromised by short-term needs to use heroin to keep the pain of withdrawal symptoms at bay.

Since people 'exist in time' their interest in autonomy must be considered over time. Individuals' interest in present pleasure may not be consistent with either their long-term autonomy or their long-term pleasure.

Autonomy is important insofar as it distinguishes humans from most animals, from 'brutes'; to deny an individual's autonomy is to treat that person as less than human. If autonomy is valued, are people committed to upholding it always in practice? Autonomy is not the only instrinsically valued concept, and there are conditions where another rule, (for example, 'not harming others') may take precedence. Current choice may compromise future choice, and arguments for long-term versus short-term autonomy must be considered. Lastly, current choice may not be autonomous, in that simply 'choosing' does not mean, by definition, that such choice is autonomous. The choice may be made without full knowledge of choices and outcome; it may be made on the basis of irrational ideas or untrue information, or the person may make the choice while in a state of mind described by others as 'not competent'.

PATERNALISM

No discussion of autonomy is possible without also considering paternalism, since this concept is often used to legitimize infringements of another's autonomy, supported as it is by the principle of beneficence. Paternalistic behaviour usually means acting on behalf of another person, in their best interest. Thus Downie and Calman (1987) describe paternalism as: 'the protection of individuals from self-inflicted harm, in the way that a mother or father looks after children'. Lindley (1988) suggests that paternalistic behaviour has two components:

1. The agent is motivated by respect for the person who is the intended beneficiary of the act.
2. The will of this person (that is, his or her current overall preference) is either disregarded or overridden by the agent.

Although paternalism is usually viewed as restricting a person's actions, this is not always the case. A person may be told a 'white lie' (paternalistic deception) in order to make them feel better, but which has no impact on action (leaving aside the question whether to 'feel worse' is an action). Lindley argues that to describe paternalism simply as 'limiting action' is too restrictive.

The dilemma posed by beneficence is thus: are there circumstances in which paternalism is justified, or does the autonomous will of the individual always take precedence? If paternalism is justified, then what are the circumstances which allow it?

Mill (1859) believed that paternalistic behaviour was never justified:

The object of this Essay is to assert one very simple principle, as entitled to govern absolutely the dealings of society with the individual in the way of compulsion or control, whether the means used be physical force in the form of legal penalties, or the moral coercion of public opinion. That principle is, that the sole end for which mankind are warranted, individually or collectively, in interfering with the liberty of action of any of their number, is self-protection. That the only purpose for which power can be rightfully exercised over any member of a civilized community, against his will, is to prevent harm to others. His own good, either physical or moral, is not a sufficient warrant. He cannot rightfully be compelled to do or forbear because it will be better for him to do so, because it will make him happier, because, in the opinion of others, to do so would be wise or even right. These are good reasons for remonstrating with him, but not for compelling him, or visiting him with any evil in case he does otherwise. To justify that, the conduct from which it is desired to deter him must be calculated to produce evil to some one else. The only part of the conduct of any one, for which he is amenable to society, is that which concerns others. In the part which merely concerns himself, his independence is, of right, absolute. Over himself, over his own body and mind, the individual is sovereign.

Despite this very forceful declaration against paternalism (and in defence of autonomy) Mill's next paragraph excludes children and those 'who are still in a state to require being taken care of', and such exclusions are discussed later.

By prohibiting the employment of paternalism it is possible that behaviour which protects autonomy might be protected. Autonomy has been discussed as existing over time, and that on occasion, short-term autonomy must give way to preserve long-term autonomy. In such instances paternalistic behaviour may operate in favour of the future, rather than the present.

In the sections on consent and competency full autonomy only exists where there is full knowledge. Since this often does not exist, paternalism may prevail in some instances — for example, where information cannot be given, either because of time or because of a person's fixed, false belief (Fadden and Fadden, 1977).

Carers very often have a strong allegiance to principles of beneficence and non-malfeasance rather than autonomy. In a discourse on ethics and clinical research, autonomy 'is not the only ethical imperative that should be considered, and perhaps an exaggerated regard for this single principle will put at risk not only the practice of scientific medicine but the whole concept of the doctor-patient relationship. Traditionally the duty of doctors is to do their best for their individual patients and not just to provide a list of alternatives from which the patients (now the consumer) select according to their needs and desires' (Baum *et al.*, 1989).

Although to prohibit actions taken in the name of beneficence may lead to harm befalling some people, so too can unrestrained paternalism cause harm by diminishing autonomy. Paternalism in health and social service personnel can lead to the denial of autonomy they should be seeking to promote. 'Killing with kindness'; may be positively motivated, but it is killing nonetheless. By doing too much for people it is possible to erode their will, and to change them subtly as an individual or prevent their development. Children need to learn through doing things for themselves and making mistakes; so too do people with learning difficulties. Over-protection and over-intrusiveness can contribute to relapse in people with schizophrenia (Leff, 1976). In such cases what is in the person's best interest does not equate with the family view of commonsense kindness.

What is best for the care team should not become what is best for the clients. People who are in quiet control may look 'happier' than disruptive people, and certainly may be easier to care for, but being quiet and controlled is not necessarily in the person's best interest.

Without the concept of paternalism, there are occasions when unnecess-ary harm would come to people, sometimes self-inflicted. The justified use of paternalism should be set against the erosion of will and personality from unchecked paternalism, and a careful set of moral checks and bal-ances weighed when arguing against autonomy, and for paternalism.

PRESCRIPTIONS FOR MENTAL HEALTH

Respect for the autonomous person implies respect for both that person's goals, and for his or her own way of pursuing them (assuming they do not infringe the autonomy of others). We can assume that most people want to be healthy, both physically and mentally, although their pursuit of this end is not always wholehearted, and may be abandoned tempor-arily in favour of short-term pleasures. If, given the exceptions mentioned above, a person's autonomy is maximized, then a concept such as 'normal' should be questioned when applied to human behaviour or mental health. And if it does, does this matter, if the 'greater good' is served?

The concept 'normal' may limit self-determination through rules and values, which might be seen as self-government. In physical health, 'normal' can be equated with 'healthy', as in 'normal temperature'. A temperature which is either too high or too low will be indicative of illness or dysfunction in the body. Can 'normal behaviour' be defined with the same confidence as definitions of 'normal temperature'?

One difference is that temperature is not under voluntary control, whereas behaviour usually is (begging questions of conditioning, and repression). Temperature can be measured objectively and the conse-quences of an abnormal temperature are also objective and measurable. Thus there is agreement, both within and between cultures, about what constitutes 'normal temperature'. Can the same be said for 'normal behaviour'?

The answer to this is no, and in any culture that passes for 'normal' is, better described as 'average'. Given differences in habits, and social norms between cultures, there is no 'overwhelming' reason to believe that 'aver-age' and 'normal' are, by definition, the same thing. If people do not know objectively what 'normal' is, then people can only judge behaviour by the value a culture puts on that behaviour, or by how well a person lives within (that is conforms to) the norms of that culture. Mental health can be only defined generally — and even then it is often negative, 'not ill' or 'not pathological'.

'Mental state utilitarianism might argue for the maximization of pleasure or happiness, but does this imply that only those who are happy or experiencing pleasure are mentally healthy? Rational-emotional therapy (Ellis, 1962) might look as though it is prescribing negative emotions but is presenting a choice. Certain irrational beliefs or ways of thinking, by their very nature, will lead to negative emotions or unhappy states. Those people who want to maximize positive emotions or happiness can challenge these irrational beliefs, and, by altering their attitudes and expectations, maximize pleasure. People who do not want to give up their irrational beliefs, (many of them actively supported by current cultural pressures) must then face the loss of pleasure (exhibited by increased anxiety, insecurity) that is a necessary consequence of holding such beliefs.

The self-determining and self-governing aspects of autonomy may be at odds with one another here. A person may want to be self-determining by promoting happiness and may see the best way of doing this as being accepted in society and conforming to its rules and beliefs. If some of these beliefs, taken to their extremes of logical progression, then cause the person unhappiness, are they not in a classic double bind? And should this not, at least according to some theorists (Bateson *et al.*, 1956), lead to mental health problems?

The arguments here become fairly tortuous as there are so many variables to take into account, so many exceptions to admit, that presenting an elegant thesis becomes close to impossible. The generalities of one argument give way to the specifics of a particular case.

Conforming to society's norms may bring some negative emotions, but at the same time 'pleasure', through acceptance. For example, society as a whole may move away from the macho mores that have held sway for so long. In some subsections of the culture however these are still the prevailing rules of behaviour. Amongst the last bastions of the machismo culture are the police, the military and fire services. In such groups, the expression of emotion is not valued, and admitting one had problems in coping would usually be seen as admitting to personal weakness:

> . . . I think there is a danger of losing something which I regard as a major British characteristic reflected in the British police — the old stiff-upper-lip if you like to call it that . . .
>
> (BBC *Horizon* television programme. Chief Supt. Bob Wells, in *Police Stress: The John Wayne Syndrome*).

Although people from the emergency and rescue services are also victims in a disaster (Raphael, 1986), and may develop post-traumatic stress disorder, the culture may resist acknowledging this. The individual in a culture which does not admit to such problems is thus doubly troubled. The rules of the culture very often take precedence, particularly if the individual wants to remain in that culture (and, if it is an occupational culture, gain promotion) to the detriment of the individual's needs. Self-government by chosen values is in opposition to self-determination; the need to express emotion is healthy for the individual.

The definition of mental health depends very much on the culture in which the individual lives, and although different philosophies and psychological theories may approve certain patterns of behaviour above others, the true essence of the human condition remains very much a matter of faith. Any approach to promoting one pattern of behaviour over another is beset by ethical dilemmas (Atkinson, 1990).

If people have the right to conform to a set of values they put above the satisfaction of their individual desires, then people also have the right not to conform. This can be taken to mean they have the right to put their own desires and wishes before the rules of the society to which they belong, although they must also suffer the consequences of this. Such consequences will usually reflect the seriousness, or otherwise, of the conventions rules or laws that have been transgressed. Distance from the behaviour also influences the way in which it is labelled. Irregular verbs abound in the field of mental health, thus:

- I'm creative;
- You're eccentric;
- He's weird.

People who do not keep peace with their companions, who chose to step to a different drummer, may well live happy, contented lives by their own standards, but be seen by others, more conventional in outlook, as living lives that are less than optimal. No one can argue that not only Henry David Thoreau lived an unconventional life in terms of his contemporaries, but also he lived a life true to his own ideals and satisfying to his beliefs. These ideals and beliefs were set down for others to read, understand and follow, if they so wished (Thoreau, 1854). His disdain for unnecessary material possessions was, however, viewed as, at best, eccentric by many of his contemporaries.

The person who chooses his or her own way can do so only at the cost of being deemed slightly odd by others. This is not, however, always the case. Sometimes the autonomy of one individual threatens the autonomy of another, or even the stability of society. To protect the individual's autonomy, within defined limits, society imposes norms of behaviour on its members. In the most permissive range, compliance brings with it acceptance, social esteem, social status and material rewards. At its most prescriptive, norms are enforced through legislation, and definitions of criminal or 'ill' behaviour.

MENTAL HEALTH PROBLEMS

In an effort to avoid stigmatizing labels such as 'mentally ill', there has been a trend to refer to people simply as having 'mental health problems'. This is seen as less stereotyping of people and thus potentially less damaging. It may be true on one social level, but less helpful in tackling some of the other issues involved. The expression 'mental health problems' covers a wide range of behaviour, from the grossly disturbed person at one extreme to the unhappy, ineffective, not coping at the other. It is this range of behaviour which itself contributes to some of the difficulties in defining appropriate responses to such behaviour. Just as response to an abnormal temperature will depend on how far it deviates from the norm, (the more extreme, the more seriously it is viewed) so behaviour which is more extreme is likely to be viewed more seriously.

Anyone who draws attention to themselves by their behaviour will face social labelling and stigmatizing; the more extreme the behaviour, the more censorious the label. Anti-psychiatrists including Laing (1960, 1967) and Szasz (1962, 1979) have argued that diagnosing such behaviour as 'ill' is simply legitimizing a social label. The argument over the veracity or otherwise of 'mental illness' (*sic*), has raged for many years. There are some people however whose behaviour causes problems.

For some it will only cause themselves problems, and such people are able to seek advice/help/treatment as they see fit. The behaviour of others causes both themselves and other people a problem. Such individuals are also free to seek advice/ help/treatment, although they may come under some pressure from family/friends/employers/society to do so. In some cases, this pressure may be institutionalized, for example when a person's probation is contingent on him for her receiving treatment. For a third group of people, the problem with their behaviour lies in its perception by (and its effect on) others. Such individuals are unlikely to seek help or advice and it is for such people that questions of autonomy loom largest.

Not all such behaviour will be labelled 'ill'. Noisy neighbours may be annoying, even extremely disruptive, but they are unlikely to be defined as 'ill' on that behaviour alone. Some behaviour, however, will be defined ill, and the more it is unlike 'normal' behaviour or experience, the more likely it will be defined as 'ill'. Thus hearing things which no-one else does, believing things no-one else does, feeling oneself to be controlled by something outside oneself are not deemed 'normal' experience, and, in the absence of any other explanation (for example drugs) may be labelled 'ill'.

Some circumstances may produce other labels ranging from mystical or religious, to acceptable, depending on context, culture and the number of people who have the same experience (Leff, 1988). Hallucinations, particularly visual, are common in bereaved people, sometimes for years after the loss (Rees, 1971) and thus in this context may be deemed 'acceptable' or 'normal'. The condition surrounding the display of some behaviour may be strict, with the implicit or explicit assumption that in other circumstances such behaviour may be seen as ill. Thus in respect of the gift of speaking in tongues, St. Paul says:

> If therefore the whole church be come together in one place, and all speak with tongues, and there come in those that are unlearned, or unbelievers, will they not say that ye are mad?
>
> (I Corinthians 15, v.23)

Does calling unusual behaviour 'ill' make a difference to the individual and their autonomy? In many ways the answer must be yes, although giving it another label may not admit autonomy. Thus although Laing speaks of the behaviour of the person labelled schizophrenic as being a 'breakthrough' rather than a breakdown. The ego is not 'the servant of the divine, no longer its betrayer' (Laing, 1967). Szasz (1974) admits to the difficulty of living with the behaviour of some people labelled 'schizophrenic'. His suggestion is, however, that such behaviour should be treated in the same way as other nuisance behaviour, by the due process of law.

The view of the reader in respect to the existence of 'mental illness' (*sic*) will influence their response to the issues raised in this chapter. Some people may have a mental health problem that can be defined as 'illness' and other people with emotional, behavioural or interpersonal problems may not be 'ill' in the accepted sense. The term 'patient' defines a particular role in relation to the doctor and health services. Many of the issues refer to all patients, not just those with mental health problems. Other terms, such as 'client', could be used where appropriate, but the term still defines someone with a 'problem', in relation to someone who expects to do something about that problem.

Much of medical ethics centres around a patient's rights, which effectively has to do with a patient's autonomy. Treatment of patients, in its broadest sense, should reflect respect for the autonomous person, which assuming the role of patient should not deny. Areas of particular importance include confidentiality, the principle of informed consent and inseparable from this, the right to refuse treatment, and competency.

CONFIDENTIALITY

Whatever, in connection with my professional practice or not in connection with it, I see or hear in the life of men, which ought not to be spoken abroad, I will not divulge, as reckoning that all should be kept secret.

(Oath of Hippocrates)

Since ancient times, confidentially has been explicit in the practice of medicine, and normally taken to mean that what a patient tells their doctor remains confidential to that relationship. This is usually extended to include other members of the multidisciplinary team who are concerned with treating the whole patient. In the age of computer-held records, patients must extend this trust further. Patients are sometimes surprised by the number, and variety, of people who have access to information about them. Downie and Calman (1987) discuss levels of information which might influence decisions about the sharing of information. It is generally assumed that information is shared between members of the team 'in the patient's best interest', that is, to facilitate care and treatments. In other cases, the sharing of information may serve another purpose, for example, in teaching. Although patients do have the right to refuse to be seen by students, many feel bound to do so, and may even have pressure put on them to agree. When this pressure comes from a medical consultant treating them they may (legitimately or otherwise) feel they will be compromising their own treatment if they continue to refuse.

Other people who are not members of the multidisciplinary care team may want information about the patient. The most common group are relatives, and may also include friends. Whilst people may be wanting information out of genuine concern for the patient, the release of information should only occur when authorized by the patient. In some circumstances, when the patient is deemed not competent, either mentally (discussed later) or practically (for example, if they are unconscious), then the next-of-kin will be given information and be asked to act on behalf of the patient and give consent. Relatives who act as carers may feel they require information about the patient to care competently for them: this will be discussed later.

Sometimes a patient's behaviour may have severe consequences for other members of the family. How far does a doctor (or other professional) have a duty to protect others at the expense of patient confidentiality? The genetic implications of certain conditions are an important area. Most people would agree that such information should be given to family members so they are able to make informed decisions, not just for themselves but with respect to unborn generations. 'Dangerousness to others' is usually taken as the major exception to the rule of confidentiality.

Recently, the Court of Appeal dismissed a claim by a patient of breach of confidentiality when a psychiatrist passed on a Report commissioned by the restricted patient's solicitors to the Director of the mental hospital and the Home Office. This was done after the patient's application to a

Mental Health Review Tribunal for conditional discharge was withdrawn after seeing the Report. The decision was that the 'balance of public interest clearly lay in the restricted disclosure of vital information to the Director of the hospital and to the Secretary of State, who had the onerous duty of safe-guarding public safety' (Dyer, 1989).

Many of the issues of confidentiality are highlighted in the famous case heard in the California Courts, now known as the 'Tarasoff decision' (Tarasoff, 1974). In this case, a young man told his therapist of his intention to kill his girlfriend. The therapist consulted with two psychiatrists and notified the police, who detained the man. He denied any intention of violence to his girlfriend and was released. He left treatment with his therapist as a result of this breach of confidence. Two months later the young man killed his girlfriend. Both the therapist and his psychiatrist-supervisor were sued by the girl's parents for failure to inform them of the patient's intent to kill their daughter.

The decision of the courts was effectively that the privilege of confidentiality and individual protection ends when the public is put at risk.

This decision has been challenged by mental health professionals. Gurevitz (1977) objects on the grounds that this decision argues in favour of psychiatry as an agent of social control, by allying the psychiatrist with a public which needs protection, rather than the need to treat an individual patient. As Gurevitz points out, most psychiatrists recognize the crucial balance of these functions and usually seek to fulfil both requirements.

One important issue is professional expertise in predicting dangerousness and the practical consequences of breaking confidentiality in such circumstances. Thus Roth and Meisel (1977) suggest that professionals are not capable of accurately predicting dangerousness. This gives rise to practical issues. Where is the threshold at which one warns possible victims? Not only does a lowering of the threshold compromise confidentiality, but might also compromise treatment. The patient may leave the therapist, indeed may leave treatment altogether, which may compromise his or her mental health, or if they do enter treatment elsewhere may conceal important information. Dangerousness may also increase, possibly because of a sense of betrayal. If this happens at the same time that treatment stops, the consequences, as in this case, may be disastrous. If confidentiality is broken, and no violence result, then the doctor may be sued by the patient for invasion of privacy or defamation of character.

Roth and Meisel have a number of practical solutions to this dilemma, including obtaining permission from the patient to warn the victim, and relying 'on odds' that violence is rare and thus not warning potential victims. Patients should be advised of boundaries surrounding confidentiality, and examining the social means of reducing the likelihood of decreasing violence (without breaking confidentiality).

In some cases, the dilemma may not be danger to other people but danger to self. Relatives may need to be given information if they are to prevent someone from harming him/herself. Relatives may also be able to give information concerning a patient's condition, for example over failure to take medication, or talk of suicide or self-harm, which may otherwise be denied by the patient. If confidentiality is preserved to the extent that doctors do not talk to relatives, such exchange is prevented.

The disclosing of information about patients as a result of being questioned by the police or being subpoenaed by the courts will vary from country to country depending on the demands of the law. Even within the law the issue, in many cases, is far from clear.

INFORMED CONSENT

Informed consent is often only raised as an issue when it is accompanied by 'determining a person's competency'. For consent to treatment, or refusal of treatment to be valid the person must both be able to understand what has been explained, and able to make their views known adequately. Consent and its relationship to law, medicine and ethics is a wide-ranging issue (Hirsch and Harris, 1988). Competency will be discussed in the next section; in this section issues of consent are discussed where the person is deemed competent.

'Consent' is the giving of permission to someone to do something which that person would not have the right to do without such permission. Thus in medicine anything which is done to the patient requires consent. Often consent is taken as 'implied; because a patient does not actively object to a procedure. Informed consent puts further strictures on the obtaining of permission, in that a patient must be able to make an 'informed' decision on the basis of evidence presented to him or her. There is a debate of how far it is possible to actually tell a patient everything, in terms of possible outcomes of every option available, and whether or not in some circumstances this can be harmful. The relevance of consent is respect for the autonomous person. Consent means that the person is allowed to exercise his or her right to determine what treatment is acceptable under what conditions, for how long and to what ends.

It is common in psychiatry for many patients to find that initial assessment of a problem merges into treatment, without the latter ever being defined, and so the patient has been given no clear opportunity to agree to treatment, or to refuse. Where patients' find themself in such a position, and are unhappy about the treatment they are receiving, they either have to challenge the doctor directly, which in itself may be very threatening, or default on treatment and run the risk of being defined as 'unco-operative' or 'poorly motivated' with all the attendant problems this may bring. This can be a particular problem for patients who do not want to take drugs, but who want to remain in the care of the psychiatrist, or remain in hospital.

It is not just methods which are not outlined, but also goals of psychotherapy may be ill-defined, and the patient may not be sure of the eventual desired outcome. A recent American review (Karasu, 1986) counted more than 400 different psychotherapies on offer. The sheer impossibility of outlining all these techniques, their rationales and underlying theories and philosophies to each and every patient, is clear, but with such a variety available, patients may not always know what is happening. That the NHS does not offer such a wide selection, does not always make the situation clearer. The fact that patients are not paying for treatment may make it easier for them to find themselves in a treatment not of their own choosing, and with little understanding of what is going on, because there was never a clear point at which they committed themselves to treatment.

If a patient has a right to consent or agree to treatment, then for autonomy to exist the converse must be true; the patient has the right to refuse treatment. Refusing treatment will, in many instances, bring with it the automatic investigation of competency. The argument simply stated, is:

– rational people want to be well;
– treatment will make the person well;
– therefore the rational person will consent to treatment.

Thus, by definition, the refusal of treatment means the person is not rational. This might be true in some cases, but for autonomy to exist, a person can both be rational and refuse treatment.

If 'well' is defined as 'socially acceptable' or 'socially conforming' then individuals may find themselves in the position of saying this goal or outcome is unacceptable to them, and they prefer their own current 'ill' behaviour. The respect for the autonomous person means accepting that people have the right to live what others may define as 'less than optimal lives' if this is their choice. Such a decision can prove very difficult for relatives to accept. They may want to act in the patient's best interest and force him or her to accept treatment. If this is not possible under the special conditions laid down in the law in the Mental Health Act, then practically (as well as legally) nothing can be done.

Such issues may be highlighted in the special case of suicide (Heyd and Bloch, 1984). This dilemma is not just differing goals (in terms of what constitutes mental health) but a disagreement over a fundamental belief — the value of life itself. It is this very denial of what is usually accepted as a universally held value that makes suicide such an emotive topic and its definition value-laden. There is no specific biblical term for killing oneself, and suicide was the term introduced as late as the 17th century to replace the more emotional and incriminatory 'self-homicide' (Daube, 1972). Until recently, killing, or attempting to kill, oneself was a crime and the successful suicide was denied burial in consecrated ground, thus underlying the belief that it was an act against the 'laws of God' as well as humankind.

In some cases suicide may be seen as a rational choice, when, for example, a patient has a terminal illness and is suffering great pain. In such cases the act is usually identified as 'euthanasia' and is outside the scope of this chapter.

Informed consent is a major issue in research in medicine. Respect for the autonomous individual is at the heart of allowing the patient to decide whether or not they want to take part in a research programme. Clinical and methodological dilemmas may be raised; consent may not always be practical or necessary (Wing, 1984; Baum *et al.*, 1989).

COMPETENCY

An individual can only be deemed to be autonomous insofar as he or she is mentally competent. Can people who are considered incompetent however be capable of autonomous choice? In many cases they can make choices. Competency operates on different levels. A person may be competent to make a wide variety of day-to-day decisions, but not competent to handle complex legal or financial affairs. Also, people who are 'mentally ill', including the dementing elderly person, may have periods when they are lucid and competent, interspersed with periods when they are not. The dilemma arises when they make choices which others consider not in their best interests, or choices which interfere with autonomy of others. In the latter case, the law may provide the answer. Both British and American law allow for the involuntary commitment of patients to a mental hospital if they are a danger to others. Although some countries, such as Italy, do not have such provision, the law can still be used to deal with antisocial behaviour which transgresses the legal code.

The decision about the competence or incompetence of a person is legal. This does not however, stop, people acting on behalf of others in many informal ways. The legal ramifications of a person being declared incompetent and the provision of 'guardians' will not be dealt with here. Benevolence is usually cited as the motivating factor in declaring someone incompetent — they can then be looked after for their own good. Even Mill has made an exception of the 'mentally ill', describing them variously as those not 'in the maturity of their faculties', 'in a state to require being taken care of by others', or those whose 'behaviour is incompatible with the full use of reflecting faculty' (Mill, 1859).

Sherlock (1986) has suggested that the current dilemma over issues such as competency stems from two revolutions in both policy and practice:

> On the one hand we are more sensitive than ever to the claims patients make for their autonomy vis-a-vis the psychiatrist and the hospital,

while at the same time our understanding of the biological roots of their illness may afford us powerful tools with which to treat them even in the absence of their consent.

It is this knowledge (or belief) in the physical causes of some 'mental illness' that affects attitudes to competency. The argument seems to be that biological changes to the brain undermine a person's autonomy, and that involuntary commitment to hospital is a rational response to someone who is no longer autonomous. By imposing treatment on a person, even if against their will, autonomy might be restored.

The same author, however, goes on to argue that: 'Even where such tools are absent the biological understanding of mental disease orients us to the way that serious mental disorder incapitiates the person against his or her will and may require care and custody even in the absence of cure' (Sherlock, 1986).

The difficulty here is if a person cannot be restored to 'the way they were' how far can society impose its norms on that person when they are no longer appropriated? Is it not possible to allow autonomy within the new framework of the person's thinking? It could be described as a new autonomy for a new biology. To deny any autonomy is to suggest that the person is now less than human. It also seems to deny any possibility of positive changes or outcomes in 'mental illness.' The reason for the changes need not be biological, but if they represent a permanent change in the person, then new rules may need to be applied. The same con-clusions might be drawn through other approaches. It could equally well be argued (in Laingian terms) of 'breakthrough' rather than 'breakdown'.

Autonomy within the incompetent (or not-as-we-define-competent) state may be allowable, but the crucial question faced by clinicians and those who formulate mental health policy and laws is, 'at what point will it be disallowed?' The arguments most frequently come back to danger-ousness — to others or to self.

What dangerousness encompasses would require at least a chapter in itself. Most people who agree that damaging another person through violent behaviour is not to be condoned, but a person's autonomy can be compromised by other aspects of the behaviour of the 'mentally ill' person, including caring for them.

At what point a person needs protection from him/herself is more open to debate. In a legal sense, 'incompetence' means that the individuals so defined are not capable of caring for themselves, their dependants or their property. The prevention of suicide or self-harm is a 'good thing', but what of the person who 'chooses' to live like a vagrant? What of the person who is prepared to risk relapse by stopping medication, because they do not like the side-effects? What of the person who is vulnerable to exploitation by unscrupulous people, who chooses to spend money in a way others consider wasteful? And at what point must such people be protected from themselves?

AUTONOMY AND SPECIAL NEEDS GROUPS

Some people are seen as 'special' in respect to autonomy: special in the sense that their right to autonomy is seen as different because of their status or condition. Children have limited autonomy because they have not yet reached maturity. John Stuart Mill was clear about this:

> Over himself, over his own body and mind, the individual is sovereign. It is, perhaps, hardly necessary to say that this doctrine is meant to apply only to human beings in the maturity of their faculties. We are not speaking of children, or of young persons below the age which the law may fix as that of manhood or womanhood. Those who are still in a state to require being taken care of by others, must be protected against their own actions as well as against external injury. For the same reason, we may leave out of consideration those backward states of society in which the race itself may be considered as in its nonage.
>
> (Mill, 1859)

Such belief is enshrined in law with parents being responsible for their children, but legal restrictions do not mean, however, that the child has fewer rights. Thirty years ago the United Nations stated that because of their vulnerability, and their innocence, children had rights over and above those of adults. The new United Nations Convention on the Rights of the Child commits governments who sign to admit globally-agreed child welfare rights into their laws. There are forty-one rights, under three headings: survival, protection and development. Discussion of this outwith the scope of a chapter on mental health, but all can be seen as bearing on both autonomy and health.

Mill was unequivocal on the rights of the child:

> It still remains unrecognised, that to bring into existence without a fair prospect of being able, not only to provide food for its body, but instruction and training for its mind, is a moral crime, both against the unfortunate offspring and against society; and that if the parent does not fulfil this obligation, the State ought to see if fulfilled, at the charge, as far as possible, of the parent.
>
> (Mill, 1859)

Since people with a mental handicap (learning difficulties) are seen as not having developed 'mental maturity' they may be treated as children. Ethical issues relating to these two groups have been addressed elsewhere (see chapter 6 by Philip Darbyshire). A paternalism exists that encourages protection from decisions people might make which are not in their own best interests, and protection from harm from others. Parents should act in the best interests of their child, and where they do not, the State should intervene on behalf of the child's interest. Recent developments like 'Childline' not only acknowledge that parents may be the source of a child's problems, but also encourage children's autonomy by giving them the means to seek help on their own behalf.

People with learning difficulties are not, however, children, no matter how much their behaviour may sometimes seem to be 'childlike'. By denying present autonomy to children we are not only protecting them in the present but we are protecting their autonomy in the future. Thus to some extent the autonomy of the adult may depend on denying autonomy to the child. Since, in the natural order of things children become adults, and spend considerably longer as adults than children, then the reasonableness of the position is seldom questioned. When, however, the position of people with a mental handicap is considered, the outcome is quite different. Although they too will mature mentally and emotionally, their development will not be the same that of as non-handicapped people. Some people will find it difficult to fit into society in a 'normal' way, either because of lack of ability, because of prejudice, or both. If such people do not have the privileges of being non-handicapped members of society, 'normal' goals or rules have limitations. Whilst it still might be reasonable to seek to protect people from harm and exploitation, other values and goals are equally valid, within their framework of reference.

The protection of the rights of children is usually seen to be a matter for the State. At the other end of the age range, protection of the rights of the elderly, particularly if they suffer from dementia, can sometimes be protected by the individuals themselves before they become incompetent. The ways in which this might be done has been discussed elsewhere (Gilhooly, 1986). The issues regarding the elderly have been set out in Chapter 5 by Barrowclough and Fleming but the loss of civil rights, or autonomy, through being declared incompetent (whether as an elderly person through dementia, or younger person through 'mental illness') can be harmful to the individual's self-esteem and psychological well-being. For people who have been intelligent, alert, productive members of society to be labelled incompetent may be a difficult stigma to bear, along with the loss of rights over self and property. Declaring someone incompetent, and appointing a guardian, is not always in the person's best interests. It may, however, be in the best interests of the person's heirs. Being declared incompetent means the person cannot amongst many other things, make or revoke a will, or otherwise manage his or her financial affairs.

It is right that children (i.e. minors under the legal age of adults) should have their rights protected; it is debatable how far adult offspring should be able to protect what they see as 'theirs', in terms of their inheritance. Some elderly people, not necessarily suffering from dementia, change the beneficiaries of their wills frequently, and on a whim. Whilst there is a possibility of unscrupulous people taking advantage, elderly individuals still have the right to deal with their money as they choose. In some countries, it is not possible to disinherit offspring totally so their rights are legally protected.

How someone chooses to spend their money when they are alive is, possibly, a different matter. If an elderly person is spending money on him/herself and enjoying it, it is unreasonable that heirs should be able to stop what they may see as 'squandering' of their inheritance.

CARERS AND AUTONOMY

In our consideration of respecting the autonomy of the person with mental health problems, scant attention has been paid to those who care for such people. Any discussion of autonomy by carers must include both formal and informal carers. Formal carers include those who are paid for caring, at any level of training. Whether caring is viewed as a job or a vocation, there is an impersonal element about it. No matter what one later feels about the person cared for, care is not motivated in the first instance by a personal relationship. Informal carers, however, are usually motivated by ties of kinship or friendship. In this respect, voluntary workers are in the first group. They might not have received payment for their caring, but it is prompted by altruism to unknown persons, rather than through a pre-existing relationship. Although many of the comments in this section apply to both formal and informal carers, there are some areas where the two groups need to be considered separately.

Both groups have certain obligations in common to the person being cared for, namely respect for their wishes, and concern for their welfare. What rights, or obligations, do carers have to themselves? Do these conflict with the rights of the patient? What happens if they do conflict?

Respect for the autonomous person includes self-development, for without this there can be no true autonomy. This applies equally to the carer and the person cared for. The moral duty to develop one's talents is found in philosophy and religious teaching from the time of Plato, Aristotle, and the Gospels. Set against this is the respect in which self-sacrifice for others is held, and which is also preached in the Gospels. The admonishment after the parable of the good Samaritan is: 'Go, and do thou likewise' (St Luke 14 v. 37) and the commandment in St John's Gospel: 'This is my commandment, That ye love one another, as I have loved you. Greater love hath no man than this, that a man lay down his life for his friend' (St John 15 v. 12–13).

The motivations of those people who choose to 'sacrifice' (*sic*) their life through caring for others are unclear, in particular the concept of vocation (Campbell, 1988). Whilst this might start as an autonomous decision such behaviours may continue for other reasons if the individuals in question have no other way of expressing themselves yet, because they have neglected all other aspects of self-development. From a purely practical point of view, even the most devoted carer must acknowledge that to care optimally means that they must fit — mentally, emotionally and physically. Downie and Calman (1987) point out that: 'there is a moral element in the most technical-seeming medical or nursing judgements'. They continue: 'If that is so, then it is important that these judgements should be the products not just of technical, scientific mind, but of a humane and compassionate one. That is why it is important for the health professional to be more than just that; to be a morally developed person who happens to follow a given professional path. Self-development, is good for both its own sake and for what it gives to patients, friends and families' (Downie and Calman, 1987).

In some cases, an excess of zeal in the caring role can lead to the diminishing of autonomy for the person cared for. This has been discussed in the section on paternalism (see page 107).

The rights of carers should be considered. Although patient's rights should always take precedence, the rights of carers are too frequently ignored completely. Carers, like other members of society, have the right to protection from patients, even when the carer has given up some rights to care for that person. The management of dangerous and violent patients in hospitals frequently gives cause for concern. Although violence towards patients cannot be condoned, the difficulty of dealing with some very disruptive patients must be acknowledged.

Another issue for formal carers requiring detailed discussion is: how far does a member of a team subject his or her autonomy to that team? This is most likely to become an issue when one member's judgement is in conflict with that of other members of the team, particularly those in senior positions, who are legally or morally responsible. Do professionals have the right to deny patients access to certain forms of treatment because they do not approve of such treatment? Does someone in training have the right to refuse to learn, or carry out, particular techniques because they do not approve of them?

The rights of informal carers have probably received even less consideration than those of formal carers, even though there are as many as six million people in Britain caring for relatives (Green, 1988). Although problems are outlined in detail in many instances (Atkinson, 1986; Hicks, 1988) and the Griffith's Report (1988) suggests that more help should be given to care for their family members, little attention is paid to their rights — in any moral sense. Caring for the ill and elderly is still often seen as 'women's work' (*sic*) and 'community care' seems to be fixed to the idea that there are women at home both able and willing to care for their relatives (Finch and Groves, 1983). This view persists despite evidence to the surprising number of men who are carers (Green, 1988).

Rights of relatives are often in opposition to the rights of patients, causing problems for the professionals involved. Professionals often refuse access to relatives in the interests of patient's right, particularly confidentiality. Denying access to information can diminish their autonomy; they are not in a position to make informed choices (Atkinson and Coia, 1989).

DELIVERY OF SERVICES

The ethical dilemmas raised by respecting the autonomous person do not permit easy answers. Whilst struggling for absolute moral answers, practical solutions have to be found, to deal with the 'here and now'.

Relatives' rights and the problems posed for patient autonomy require solutions to this dilemma. They should include treating relatives as clients in their own right, and provide them with professional services of their own, provide information and education, advice and support (Atkinson and Coia, 1989).

Organisations such as World Health Organisation, World Federation for Mental Health and the World Psychiatric Association can act as guardians of ethical standards, overseeing the practice of psychiatry on a global scale. On a more local scale, the Mental Welfare Commission exists to protect the rights of patients in Britain, and every patient has the right of access to the Commission. Pressure groups such as MIND and other consumer-driven groups can also act to protect the rights of the individual, and highlight injustice and bad practice.

Changes in the way in which services are delivered can also increase the autonomy of the patient by recognizing his or her right to choose as a consumer. As a first step, with little change needed to services, patients could be given more information about their condition. Without such information, no real choices can be made (Atkinson, 1989). Although some people might object to this being done by professionals, seeing it as 'indoctrination' by powerful and traditional groups, whether people choose to stay and be treated within the system, or leave the system, they have a right to influence the behaviour of professionals.

A more radical approach is that of service brokerage, developed in Canada with people with mental handicaps (Brandon and Towe, 1989; Ney and Sone, 1988). 'Brokerage is the technical arm of an autonomous planning mechanism that is community based and consumer controlled' (Brandon and Towe, 1989).

Whatever answers advance the resolution of these dilemmas regarding autonomy and mental health, ethical reasoning must always underpin practical answers. Everyday realities however will always temper moral absolutes.

REFERENCES

Atkinson, J. M. (1986) *Schizophrenia at Home* Croom Helm, London.

Atkinson, J. M. (1989) To tell or not to tell the diagnosis of schizophrenia. *Journal of Medical Ethics*, **15**, 21–24.

Atkinson, J. M. (1990) Health education in mental health. In Doxiodis, S. (ed.) *Ethics in Health Education*. John Wiley, Chichester.

Atkinson, J. M. and Coia, D. A. (1989) Responsibility to carers — an ethical dilemma. *Psychiatric Bulletin*, **13**, 602–604.

Bateson, G., Jackson, D. D., Haley, J. and Weakland, J. (1956) Towards a theory of schizophrenia. *Behavioural Science*, **1**, 251–264.

Baum, M., Zilkha, K. and Houghton, J. (1989) Ethics of clinical research: lessons for the future. *British Medical Journal*, **299** 251–253.

Brandon, D., Towe, N. (1989) *Free to Choose. An Introduction to Service Brokerage.* Good Impressions, London.

Campbell, A. V. (1988) Profession and vocation. In Fairburn, C. and Fairburn, S. (eds.) *Ethical Issues in Caring*. Gower Publishing, Aldershot.

Daube, D. (1972) The linguistics of suicide. *Philosophy and Public Affairs*, **1**, 415–417.

Downie, R. S. and Calman, K. C. (1987) *Health Respect: Ethics in Health Care*. Faber and Faber, London.

Dyer, C. (1989) Public interest and a psychiatrist's duty of confidentiality. *British Medical Journal*, **229**, 1301.

Ellis, A. (1962) *Reason and Emotion in Psychotherapy*. Lyle Stuart, Secaucus, N. J.

Fadden, R. and Fadden, A. (1977) False belief and the refusal of medical treatment. *Journal of Medical Ethics*, **3**, 133–136.

Finch, J. and Groves, D. (1983) *A Labour of Love: Women, Work and Caring*. Routledge and Kegan Paul, London.

Gilhooly, M. L. M. (1986) Legal and ethical issues in the management of the dementing elderly. In Gilhooly, M. L. M., Zarit S. H. and Birren, J. E. *The Dementias*. Prentice Hall, New Jersey.

Green, H. (1988) *Informal Carers*. (General Household Survey 18985 GHS No 15 Supplement A). HMSO, London.

Griffiths, Sir R. (Chairman) (1988) *Community Care. Agenda for Action — A Report to the Secretary of State for Social Services*. HMSO, London.

Gurevitz, H. (1977) Tarasoff: Protective privilege versus public peril. *American Journal of Psychiatry*, **134**, 289–292.

Heyd, D. and Bloch S. (1984) The ethics of suicide. In Bloch, S. and Chodoff, P. (eds.) *Psychiatric Ethics*. Oxford University Press, Oxford.

Hicks, C. (1988) *Who Cares: Looking After People At Home*. Virago, London.

Hirsch, S. R. and Harris, J. (1988) *Consent and the Incompetent Patient: Ethics, Law and Medicine*. Gaskell, London.

Karasu, T. B. (1986) The specificity versus non-specificity dilemmas: toward identifying therapeutic change agents. *American Journal of Psychiatry*, **143**, 687–695.

Laing, R. D. (1960) *The Divided Self: A Study of Sanity, Madness and the Family*. Tavistock Publications, London.

Laing, R. D. (1967) *The Politics of Experience*. Penguin, Harmondsworth.

Leff, J. P. (1976) Schizophrenia and sensitivity to the family environment. *Schizophrenia Bulletin* **2**, 566–574.

Leff, J. P. (1988) *Psychiatry Around the Globe. A Transcultural View* 2nd ed. Gaskell, London.

Lindley, R. (1988) Paternalism and caring. In Fairburn, G. and Fairburn, S. (eds.) *Ethical Issues in Caring*. Gower Publishing, Aldershot.

Mill, J. S. (1859) *On Liberty* and (1861) *Utilitarianism* (edition quoted from, for both: *Utilitarianism*. Warnock, M. (ed.) (1969) Fontana, London.

Newton, J. (1988) *Preventing Mental Illness*. Routledge and Kegan Paul, London.

Ney, H. and Sone, O. (1988) Service brokerage. *Rehabilitation Digest*, **18**, 16–17.

Paton, H. J. (1969) *The Moral Law. Kant's Groundwork of the Metaphysics of Morals*. Hutchinson, London.

Raphael, B. (1986) *When Disaster Strikes. A Handbook for the Caring Professionals*. Hutchinson, London.

Rees, W. D. (1971) The hallucinations of widowhood. *British Medical Journal*, **iv**, 37–41.

Roth, L. H. and Meisel, A, (1977) Dangerousness, confidentiality, and the duty to warn. *American Journal of Psychiatry*, **134**, 508–511.

Sherlock, R. (1986) My brother's Keeper? Mental health policy and the new psychiatry. In Kentsmith, D. K., Salladay, S. and Miya, P. A. *Ethics in Mental Health Practice*. Grune and Stratton, New York.

Szasz, T. (1962) *The Myth of Mental Illness*. Secker and Warburg, London.

Szasz, T. (1979) *Schizophrenia*. Oxford University Press, Oxford.

Tarasoff vs. the Regents of the University of Calfornia (1974) 118 *California Reporter*. **129**, 529, p 2d 553.

Thoreau, H. D. (1854) *Walden*. (Rpt. 1951) Hendrick House, New York.

Townsend P. and Davidson N. (1982) *Inequalities in Health*. Penguin, Harmondsworth.

Wing, J. K. (1984) Ethics and psychiatric research. In Bloch, S. and Chodoff, P. (eds.) *Psychiatric Ethics*. Oxford University Press, Oxford.

Chapter Eight

The consequences of service planning in mental health nursing

MARTIN WARD

EDITORS' INTRODUCTION

Traditionally, mental health services have been channelled through psychiatric nurses, although their actual function has never been clear. The role of psychiatric nurses as 'handmaidens', or mere supports, to the expression of medical treatment is little more than an historical fact. Psychiatric nurses have begun to take themselves, and their role as service providers, seriously. At least part of this change of emphasis involves a reflection on past values and present committments. Psychiatric nurses cannot be expected to provide unilateral services. Although psychiatric nurses may represent the major medium of 'care', the contributions of other professional groups will serve to clarify their own definition.

The sheer size of the professional grouping of psychiatric nurses sets them apart from all other service providers. In this chapter **Martin Ward** considers how such a large resource might be used 'properly'. Nurses have been used in the past as the means of restricting the lifestyles of people with mental health problems. As psychiatric nurses try to forge a new role for themselves, who will acknowledge the humanity of those in their care, what ethical problems are likely to emerge?

The consequences of service planning in mental health nursing

One of the greatest problems faced by most practising psychiatric nurses is the lack of control they have over what takes place within the care environment. Because legal responsibility rests with senior medical staff, it is they who determine the direction, style and objectives of care input (Keddy, 1985). Their role however dictates that they may have minimal client contact, seldom undertake therapy, and are often unaware of the methodology required to produce it. In effect, this creates a dichotomy between the two main disciplines in psychiatry, namely medicine and nursing. The first, whose primary function has been refined to diagnosis and the provision of physical methods of care, determines the actions of the second, whose primary function is essentially the provision of practical help. Placed against a backdrop of client needs and expectations, it is not too difficult to conjure a situation where all three of these groups have opposing views on the purpose and direction of individualized psychiatric help, with a resultant dilution of effectiveness.

Such a situation raises serious questions about the ethical nature of professional decision-making and its subsequent effects on the influence of both nursing and its recipients. For, as Jameton (1984) indicated, it is during care planning that all ethical stances must be tested against the problem in question, in an attempt to establish the best. This cannot be achieved in a climate designed to exclude ethical alternatives.

If a more effective ethical framework with an inherent practical intent is to be established, it becomes necessary to examine in detail the key areas of care planning, the roles and philosophies of those involved, and the desired outcomes of modern psychiatric intervention. Before doing so however, some understanding is required of the ethical theories associated with care provision. In short, it is a question of who is doing what, and why?

WHO DOES WHAT?

Raatikainen (1989) explored the possibility of how the scientific and technological advances made within nursing, might, when mixed with ordinary human values, affect nurses' abilities to provide compassionate and benign intervention. The advances referred to were not so much the methods of delivering physical forms of care, but more the actual mechanics of nursing, such as its philosophy, and those elements that created client emancipation, individualized care and an enlightened and scientific approach to clinical performance. This has tremendous significance for psychiatric nurses, because although one should not draw universal generalizations from specific situations (Trusted, 1979), it is in the area of attitudes, philosophies and professional roles that the ethical nature of nursing bears most scrutiny (Bottorff and D'Cruz, 1984).

Nurses, and particularly psychiatric nurses, have long geared their practice towards a humanistic perspective. Increasingly, the process of care management has become a mutual activity between the nurse and the client, with both responsibility and accountability shared equally. This humanistic quality demands freedom of expression, real decision-making activities, and in many circumstances the 'right to be wrong'. There is almost a collusion between nurses and their clients working together to get what is best for the client. This approach to nursing with its dependence upon such human qualities as respect, empathy, goodness and trust, is somewhat out of step with modern technological advances that appear to place greater emphasis on professionalism and clinical rights.

In truth such a conclusion is fallacious because it is the belief of individual nurses about themselves, and how they should carry out their jobs, which will determine how they implement such advances into their clinical performance. If their methodology is based upon equanimity and emancipation, they will react in a fundamentally different way to those nurses whose methodology is based upon theoretical values, rights and procedures. Nursing process activities, with their inherent demands on nurses and clients alike, cannot successfully be carried out by nurses who believe that power and a professional hierarchy are an acceptable part of the clinical scene. Equally, nursing process activities cannot be fully implemented if clients are not fully aware of what is expected of them (Ward, 1985). Thus, modern advances within psychiatric nursing do not preclude what Raatikainen (1989) referred to as 'The Golden Rule' of nursing (i.e. the highest ethical principles are based upon a sense of caring when clients are at their most vulnerable).

A nurse's ethical principles should not, therefore, be compromised by changes and developments within nursing and its allied sciences; rather, they should be adapted and used to enhance those principles. It is because nurses attempt to function in such close harmony with their clients, however, that they so often find themselves diametrically opposed to the demands and wishes of other disciplines. It is this quality of humanness that enables them to experience client empathy on such a personal level, but that contradicts the more diagnostic and less involved status of such people as doctors, physiotherapists and even occupational therapists who, in theory at least, are the disciplines most closely aligned with psychiatric nurses. As a consequence, combined with their lack of real control within the clinical environment, the contracts, alliances and management routines they may have agreed with their clients, do not always take place and in some cases are simply ignored (Lebow, 1982; Shields, 1985; Shields *et al.*, 1988). This ethical situation, though not quite a 'dilemma' because it does have a solution, does fall within the broad spectrum of what Tschudin (1986) has called 'normative', or 'prescriptive' ethics, or, what *should* happen, but doesn't always.

NORMATIVE AND DESCRIPTIVE ETHICS

To understand the significance of this situation, and to see how it might affect the ability of a nursing practitioner to develop serious care planning strategies, traditional nursing and medical positions should be viewed from an ethical standpoint. It would be too much to say that doctors and nurses do not think the same way, but their expectations of clinical practice are certainly at variance with each other.

The basis of this assumption stems from the ethical standpoints traditionally associated with the two disciplines. Nurses, who tend to be more patient-orientated, have tended to use an ethical approach known as 'normative' or 'prescriptive'. This is mainly a philosophical and subjective approach, which places emphasis on recommendations for the way people should behave. It concerns itself with codes of conduct, rights and principles, and addresses the problems of human suffering, compassion, and the concepts of care. Doctors, however, have traditionally used another ethical approach known as descriptive, or scientific. This approach is concerned with making sense of behaviour, through observation and investigation, so that statements can be made on an objective level. It is less concerned with sociological or subjective factors and places significance on physical and psychological expressions of behaviour.

Even a casual discussion on the two approaches suggests that they are very different. Doctors tend to diagnose (a scientific activity), while nurses tend to deliver care, often a subjective pursuit. Doctors make decisions concerning care management, which are acted upon, whilst nurses (certainly within a psychiatric setting) discuss various managerial and clinical possibilities over which they have little executive control. The doctor will describe how a person will receive electro-convulsive therapy, the nurse will discuss whether the patient should receive it or not. The doctor decides what will happen, the nurses what ought to happen.

Largely as a result of medical dominance within the health care setting, nurses have assumed a secondary role consistent with their ethical standpoint. In psychiatry, this causes serious clinical problems, which ultimately cannot be resolved unless nurses alter their traditional stance. Problems, such as decision-making, problem tackling, therapy directives, negotiation, clinical management and care delivery, are all the products of modern technological changes. Nurses have generated this new and exciting environment but need to be aware of its ramifications if they are to become effective practitioners within it.

ETHICAL INFLUENCES

Before considering the practicalities of ethical changes upon nursing care management there are two other elements that must be brought into the equation. First, and perhaps most significant of all, is the person him or herself, and second the relationship of an ethical approach, such as normative, or descriptive ethics, when considered against a backdrop of ethical theory.

The client

The person's ethical approach to self-preservation, safety and self-determination may well be seen as complementary to that of the nurse, yet it is not uncommon to find the less demanding psychiatrist seen as the safer object by the client. Could it be that clients' expectations of medical staff lead them to believe that they, and only they, will be able to help them because of their controlling influence and scientific approach? Nurses get just a 'little too close' to the problem because of their working relationship and constant contact, and are therefore too much of a threat. Because nurses are able to get close to their clients, the clients view them as being as vulnerable as themselves and therefore in no real position to actually help them?

When clients are asked to decide between the decisions of medical or nursing staff, their natural inclination is to select those which appear to be the most positive, though not always those decisions which are the most helpful.

For real care planning to take place between nurse and clients this natural familiarity experienced by the nurses has to be overcome in some way if they are to be taken seriously by their clients. After all, it is the client who expects care by the system; the question of who gives it is not an ethical issue, but more about consumer demand. Nurses have got to present themselves as viable alternatives to other disciplines within the care environment, without losing the human values, without prejudicing their ethical approach, yet with the introduction of positive professional action designed to bring about therapeutic change.

Ethical theory

Ethical theories come under two separate groups: those which observe a situation, then try to predict its consequences and choose options that will provide the greatest good for those involved; and those which observe the situation, list the relevant rights, claims and principles of that situation or individual, and then select the option which serves justice best. These two groups are known as **consequentialism** and **non-consequentialism** respectively (Thiroux, 1980).

Consequentialism, based on utilitarianism, represents the 'greatest happiness' principle, whereby behaviour options are chosen because the individual is predicted as benefitting most on a personal level. Nurses may decide that such an approach best suits clinical identity, and their traditional ethical approach may well complement such an approach. In doing so however it will also reinforce the person's belief that the nurse is really not the agent of change, but simply a good friend and supporter. This is hardly the right approach needed for constructive psychiatric nursing. Other views exist, however (Clarke; Baldwin and Barker, this volume).

Non-consequentialism attempts to resolve moral dilemmas by considering the action that will be needed to do so. In effect it is not totally concerned with subjective feeling or responses, and as a result tends to be arbitrary in its decision-making processes. Given that medical staff often use decision-making skills based upon a person's rights and principles (and that these are often recognized by patients as being desirable qualities in a care giver) then perhaps nurses might need to adopt a non-consequential stance if they are to be taken more seriously, or even recognized as alternatives to their medical colleagues.

The dilemma here is that the natural sense of justice which prevails in most nurses does not always extend to justice, regardless of the consequences. For example, what good is it organizing community support, community psychiatric nurse (CPN) visits, social work and social services follow-ups if the person commits suicide on the way home in the taxi? There has to be, however, some rapprochement of the ethical theories if nurses are to be allowed to practice both ethical approaches to care delivery, with all their attendant human virtues, whilst somehow converting their desire for justice into a more humanistic and consequential direction.

Morrison (1989) considered this problem, but from another angle, when he suggested that some nurses' perception of themselves did not match that which they felt a professional nurse should be. In fact all of Morrison's respondents felt that self-improvement was necessary, thus demonstrating that many nurses were both unhappy, and unsure of their clinical role, their relationships with fellow professionals and their clinical achievements. The question needs to be asked: if nurses are unhappy with themselves, are the clients for whom they care also dissatisfied with them?

Within the realms of ethical theory and approach the answer is probably 'no', for most clients are close enough to their nurses to feel that they are too similar to be really effective. In terms of being a consumer and demanding an effective service, however, the answer might well be a resounding 'yes'. After all, what is the point in having several different professional groups caring on your behalf when one of those groups appears to make little or no executive decisions, is seldom seen as being in control whilst in the company of the discipline members, and is unwilling or unable to make care decisions until they have been sanctioned by others. If a person merely required a professional 'friend' they would ask their next-door neighbour to do the job; but some might see that as taking the analogy a little too far.

If nurses are to come to terms with their own ethical position and deliver a successful service which enables others to develop equally, then such practicalities have to be explored. There are ten areas that form the key to the application of ethical theory within a psychiatric nursing setting. They are as follows.

1. Who **controls** care planning? What does the person do?
2. How does the person get to **express** her/himself within the care plan?
3. How many **mistakes** (i.e. decisions or choices, which are subsequently altered) can a person make on a care plan?
4. How **legal** is total care emancipation?
5. What will happen to psychiatry if institutions maintain their current control of care?
6. How do current philosophies of psychiatric nursing differ from those of the traditional institution, and what are the implications of such a situation?
7. Are nurses going to **assert** themselves?
8. How much **communication** is needed for item 7 to occur and, what effect will that have on person-orientated strategies?
9. Do nurses actually **need** to change?
10. Who is going to make the **decisions** in the future?

CARE PLANNING AND ITS CONTROL

Care planning takes place on two levels. If one ignores the mechanics of nursing for a moment and looks at the processes at work, certain behaviours are clearly expected of certain individuals. Nurses, clients and other members of the multi-disciplinary team all have a specific part to play and yet seldom does anyone identify that role. For example, nurses expect their clients to be stressed, unhappy, dissatisfied, frightened, angry, and disorientated, so they tend to adopt their supportive, yet slightly defensive, attitude towards them. This expectation seems logical: if patients were fully competent there would be little point in becoming a patient. The nurse has assumed a level of client competence that may, or may not, be reinforced during the course of their clinical relationship. From an ethical standpoint, this could be seen as initiating the normative approach — therapeutic protection.

Conversely, the client has his or her expectations of the nurse who will be strong, supportive, intelligent, but caring, sympathetic, knowledgeable, unflappable and young. As a consequence of such ideas the client will expect behaviours of the nurse equally as positive, though many clients still see nurses as being in a subordinate role and are disturbed by their unfamiliar assertiveness.

This is the beginning of the first level of care planning, setting the scene, establishing the roles, clarifying positions and trying to reinforce expectations. This first level progresses to the point where both nurse and client try to fit each other into their set patterns. If they are successful, such stereotyping will ultimately produce stagnant care planning, because neither expects much of the other. If they are unsuccessful, then it is because either client or nurse has demonstrated behaviour which breaks the stereotyped pattern and may be seen by the other as threatening. It is only if preconceived ideas are challenged, however, that any real progress can be made, so of the two alternatives, this is the most suitable. Of course, the nurse should be aware of these influences and use that knowledge to clarify with the client about the progress of their relationship. The nurse's skill at keeping the person informed, while still managing to produce a climate of safety and support, will be truly tested, but such an approach is necessary if the relationship is to develop for the benefit of the person.

The second level of care planning is only completed once the first is complete. This is the process of deciding upon priorities, by establishing behavioural responses and identifying individual or group strategies. None of these can take place unless the first level is complete because if relationships, roles and social positions have not at least begun to be sorted out, they will certainly interfere with the professional caring.

Of the two levels of care planning, the first poses the most difficult ethical problem because it is often a spontaneous, even preconceived, activity. Attitudes, beliefs and social behaviours are not easy to change at the drop of a hat, and nurses are just as prone to prejudice as anyone else. If a nurse has already chosen his or her particular approach to a client, then it is difficult to see how, without some miraculous event taking place, he or she may be dissuaded from completing it. If the nurse has chosen to be forthright, assertive and strong, it is unlikely that the client will resist this approach or confront the professional. As a consequence of this, the whole of the second level of care planning will be dominated by the nurse, with the client playing a very passive, or submissive role. If, however, the nurse has chosen to be conciliatory and spontaneous, then the person may take advantage of this and reverse the situation. A dominant client may be more acceptable than a passive one, but care planning has to be a shared process for it to be truly effective. In ethical terms, it is the second, or consequential approach which ought to be adopted by the nurse, but not in its absolute form.

Control over care-planning can only be seen as a joint activity if the first level is completed in a climate of openness, high communication and responsiveness, with both clients and nurses identifying their own roles very early in the relationship. The biggest problems faced by the nurses will be to decide just what his or her perceived role actually is, how to communicate that to the client, and how, on a reciprocal basis he or she will enable clients to establish and convey back their perceived role.

The use of nursing process should facilitate this activity, but as yet it is in the area of communication that most difficulty has been experienced with this approach to care delivery (Allen, 1981; Shields, 1985; Topf, 1988). Establishing 'intent' through effective communication is not a problem unique to psychiatric nurses and their clients, but it is certainly a sad indictment of a profession whose work is based upon the interactive process that still remains such a crucial issue within the care delivery debate. Control of care delivery must be a shared activity, fully discussed and agreed by both clients and nurses (Ward, 1988).

The desire of the nurse to co-operate fully with the client's needs stems from the nurse's belief in equality and equanimity. The communication that enables the client to appreciate this fact will ultimately take place as a consequence of that belief.

Unless psychiatric nurses are taught the qualities and expressions of human values as applied to their work, and given the opportunity to express themselves in the same way as their future clients, this desired state of professional equality and person emancipation will not take place. It is an extremely resourceful and resilient nurse who is able to promote these human qualities if his or her educational programme has reduced them to the level of 'schoolchild'. The natural tendency towards morality, caring and enlightenment should be fostered by an expressive or experimental approach to professional development. Nurses, like anyone else, will only do unto other as they have been done unto themselves.

The decisions about care and control must rest with the main provider of care and its recipients. Medical staff and other professionals must honour those decisions, but nurses must take responsibility for their own actions, just as they expect their patients to do the same. The ethical issue here is not 'who should control' but 'how should the controllers control'? Education, personal belief, and clinical experience remain at the heart of the issue.

PERSONAL EXPRESSION

Nursing exists, within the UK, in a climate of the nursing process and a whole variety of nursing models. These clinical developments evolved in the USA, the nurses in Britain appear to use them for different reasons (De la Cuesta, 1983). In America the emphasis is on the professionalism of the nurse, whilst in the UK the emphasis is on the quality of the care provided. One must assume that the two approaches are not mutually exclusive, but serious ethical problems exist.

There is an alarming trend in the USA to 'scientize' psychiatric nursing so that it gains credibility. The use of coded nursing diagnosis, matrix frameworks, computer-orientated observational criteria and other such 'high-tech' devices suggests that the patients input into care is limited to the shape and form of software memory banks (Brown *et al.*, 1987; Coler and Vincent, 1987; Ehrman, 1988; Norris and Kuens-Connell, 1988). British nurses may eventually follow the trends of their North American colleagues, but in this particular area the adoption of such a philosophy would not only contradict the ethical approach of most psychiatric nurses but would also contravene the principles of the UK approach to its nursing process. Client exclusion, by scientific or any other means, is incompatible with self-expression and personal involvement.

Certainly the emphasis in the UK is one of improving the system for the clients (Brooking, 1988) rather then making the system itself more effective, despite the client. Self-expression for the client remains the only way that nurses can effectively gauge the appropriateness of their interventions, and the use of techniques such as interactive counselling, active listening, covert and overt observational skills, expressive therapies such as art, music and literature and various forms of group work remain the best way that such personal expression can be facilitated. Alternatively, citizen advocacy and self-advocacy systems can be established. The only way that nurses can establish an observational background for the provision of individualized care is through the person's own verbal or nonverbal expressions.

In elderly people, where the biological effects upon memory have created a situation which precludes orientation, the same observational activities are necessary. Self-expression does not necessarily spring from verbal ability. The skill of the nurse is in recognizing self-expression in all aspects of human behaviour and relating it to personal experience. If all psychiatric nurses adopted a totally 'scientific' approach to care-planning and implementation, they would be guilty of reducing their clients to classified factors, manipulated to suit the system, not explored in their own right. Such an approach is incompatible with the ethical values of consequentialism.

CLIENT MISTAKES

Trial and error is a recognized stage of human development. It is a process whereby children explore themselves and their environment, establish a social pattern, and above all else try to make sense of what is going on. It is an active decision-making process which, when refined to its ultimate level, can produce alternatives otherwise unthinkable. Why should a psychiatric client be denied one of the most fundamental of all decision-making activities? The simple answer is that they should not. The very nature of trial and error is most adequately suited to much of current psychiatric therapy theory. If an individual is to develop him/herself and reach full potential, he or she has to establish which elements of his or her behaviour are most suited to the desired life style and personal ethos. Self-awareness, personal development, assertiveness, confidence and control are all factors in the process of maturation. Likewise, within psychiatry, the belief that each person has the key to unlock their own personal 'skeletal cupboard' has long been accepted as a logical stance for therapists. If patients are unaware of the steps, decisions and strategies used to bring about a more satisfactory approach to their personal behaviour then they are unlikely to be able to adapt those activities to future difficulties. Some clients will need to be taught new behaviours by virtue of restricted repertoires. Others, however, do not need opportunities to learn new behaviours, but rather require a supportive context to allow established behaviours to flourish. Given the opportunity to explore those alternatives themselves and make decisions about how they should be used, devised and adapted, such individuals will have a greater understanding both of their own dynamics and competencies. This gives them a greater experiential base to work from when next confronted with personal difficulties, and they will then have the opportunity to make decisions based upon choice, not ignorance.

The process of trial and error is an inherent part of that growth, and nurses must allow clients to explore alternatives both of their own making and creativity, as well as their own choice, so that they can find out for themselves just what is appropriate or satisfying. Nurses do not have the right, especially in a climate of care-sharing, to deny patients the 'right to be wrong'. Only by exploring behaviours which are unacceptable or unsatisfying can a client ever hope to experience those which are most positive.

Within the realms of consequentialism, this forms the basis of 'the greatest happiness principle' when applied to nursing. Happiness here is decided by success. There are situations where the alternatives chosen by clients represent a threat to their own personal safety, or even to their life. Allowing a patient to take his or her own life by jumping out of a window or cutting his or her throat is anathema to professional ethics. At this stage in care-planning, control must be exerted by the nurse about the direction that the person's problem-solving takes. Suicide is an act of desperation from a lack of other perceived alternatives. The nurse should step back from this situation (as with any other life-threatening or body-abusing equivalent) and offer alternatives about the prevailing causes of the whole sequalae. The question is not about letting the person make the mistake of taking his or her own life, but exploring the rights and wrongs of decisions and actions made beforehand, which led to the ultimate expression of feeling, and made the patient choose suicide rather than some other option.

Safety factors, resources and certain social influences represent the only real factors that might preclude a client from being given the 'right to be wrong'. Nurses have to deal with their own frustrations in their own way; they should not force clients into making decisions which are expedient but ultimately self-defeating.

Of course the major dilemma for nurses in such a situation is that this process of 'allowing clients to be wrong' takes more time than teaching them how to be right, albeit without knowing why. This means that nurses must often support their clients in a more positive way, and possibly even defend them from others who expect fast results and fast turnover.

THE LEGALITIES OF EMANCIPATION

Client emancipation, the prospective refinement of the nursing process, is not a new idea (van Maanen, 1984). Each client should assume control over all care-planning decisions, including deciding about alternatives and negotiating the final cessation of care, without prejudice to the rights of quality of care input. Clients' rights within psychiatry are usually the domain of legislation which controls their freedom, not the way they exercise it. There should be no argument about a person's right to self-determination and individual dignity. In ethical terms the nurse is really not in a position to adopt a care-planning strategy which denies clients the opportunity to make decisions about what should happen to them. Consequentialism is about people finding their own level, their own happiness, their own freedom from pain, their own peace. This is not an activity that can be achieved by someone else on their behalf. There are no legal constraints to client emancipation, just a lack of imagination on the part of some unenlightened or thoughtless psychiatric nurses.

THE CONSEQUENCES OF INSTITUTIONAL CONTROL

From an ethical stance it is difficult to equate the developments that have taken place within psychiatric nursing with the traditional approach to care control exerted by the major institutions of the profession. Institutions base their control upon statutes, legislation, the manipulation of socio-political factors and financial resources. Their aims are often ruled by the limitations of those resources, and not necessarily by the desire to produce the best possible product. Their political status implies a position which is almost materialistic, in that they are dedicated to producing the best possible service within the constraints of financial limitations, as opposed to simply providing the best. They have to balance the books, whilst complying with the ground rules of the 'letter of the law'. Their approach is therefore 'non-consequentialism in nature, descriptive by design'.

This stance supports some members of the multi-disciplinary team but it is totally at variance to that of autonomous nursing practitioners. The effects of having a clinical environment manipulated by non-clinicians is difficult enough for many nurses to deal with, but the situation is exacerbated when the demands of those non-clinicians take precedence over the clinicians and is counter-productive for care planning. There are, therefore, two issues; a conflict of perceived ethical theory, and conflict of professional interest. Both will cause a breakdown in communication, arguments, wasted time, frustration, and an interruption in care-planning activities, but the eventual consequences of such a conflict can only be conjecture.

Traditionally, when management makes decisions in nursing that are disliked, or felt to be unjust, by practising nurses, an increase occurs in industrial action, non-compliance and general disruption. For various reasons, eventually, the workforce is expected to conform to the decision and continue as if nothing had happened. Nurses then show their disapproval by resigning, or simply not participating fully in the clinical role; they lose personal dignity, get angry with each other and their morale plummets.

If nurses develop their skills, identify new and exciting methods of care delivery, unite the demands of the system with the needs of the client, and generally improve the professional and civil rights of their clients, a similar situation will occur. Specifically, the implementation of unpopular or unwelcome initiatives by nurse managers may increase the probabilities of non-compliance or resignation by nurse practitioners. This would result in fewer staff to complete the new work. The staff that remain become demoralized and pressurized, and a management system that continues with its traditional stance, gradually reduce the work force, and remain oblivious that it is the cause of the original problem. Management, however, would not recognize there was a problem because managers would 'rationalize' resources as nursing staff left. As they have little knowledge of the clinical scene, they would not appreciate the increase in pressure on the remaining staff, and would expect nurses to deal with their own problems.

No one can determine what would happen if these two conflicts of interest were sorted out. Speculation concerning staff morale and shortages only produces the same feelings of frustration as the major problem itself. Nurses however have a moral and professional responsibility to act as advocates for their clients; whilst the institution retains total control over the shape and style of health care provision, the ethical dilemma that this provokes is not conducive to nursing advocacy. Nurses must assert themselves within the clinical and managerial arena, otherwise clients will not be given the opportunity to express themselves in the manner that their care dictates.

PHILOSOPHICAL CONFLICTS

The ethical dilemma faced by nurses is also apparent within the philosophical arena. The sensation of being undervalued by a governing authority and having clinical and technical skills devalued (by virtue of them being ignored) is both philosophically and ethically relevant. The philosophies of general management and collective responsibility for large groups do not equate with the individualized philosophy of a practising nurse dealing with individuals (who may or may not be within a group).

Ethically, the institutional situation demands a non-consequentialistic approach to care-delivery, which does not equate with the individual nurse trying to use a consequentialistic approach within the close confines of his or her local clinical arena. This situation applies to all psychiatric nursing staff, but especially to those working within a large infrastructure, where the power base rests firmly with other disciplines. Specialist nursing groups sometimes have an advantage, in that they have more control over which clients they choose to see and how they develop their care. Community psychiatric nurses, family therapists, and clinical nurse specialists and consultants come under this heading. They too however, can have their designs frustrated by managerial groups (out of their domain) making professional demands upon them that are not necessarily designed to improve the quality of the service, but to rationalize financial resources. Unfortunately such situations often develop into arguments about principles, rather than dealing with the real facts.

The main area of concern within these 'institution versus nursing' philosophies is that of priorities. The priority of the institution should be to provide the best possible level of care to its clients within the confines of its budget and the limitations of its human resources. Individuals are not really catered for, because if an institution has to deal with 500 people individually, not one group of 500 people, the time spent on manipulating the system to meet those individual requirements would be self-defeating. Hence the institution devises strategies that are consistent with common ground, not individuality. Unfortunately, when the nurse is placed in the situation of being the main agent of the institution, his or her own philosophical premise restricts the ability to be either a nurse or a care manager.

To understand this problem, the dimensions of the care delivery system used by the nurse should be considered. In most places within the Western world, some form of the nursing process is used by practising psychiatric nurses. Inherent within its philosophy is the belief in equality and client emancipation. If nurses are to implement this system fully, they must ensure both the clients' right to make (and carry out) care decisions. They should also fulfil the role of a nurse with responsibility for support of the patient, supervision of the care programme, and the provision of resources necessary for everyday living (i.e. food, comfort, safety). The philosophical dilemma should be quite obvious: the nurse is expected to be one thing for the client as well as something different for the institution. As the agent of the institution, the nurse is expected to support its rules and regulations. This means that nurses should both treat their clients as a group of individuals with similar problems and difficulties, and, treat those same clients as individuals with different problems and difficulties. This is an irreconcilable problem, unless one becomes dominant over the other, or if there is a degree of compromise by both parties.

For compromise to occur both parties must first admit that there is a problem to be solved. Mutual concessions are not possible if either party is unaware or unprepared to see the nature of a problem. Unfortunately, within most health care environments, as with all social groups, it is the weakest link that makes the most concessions. This is the product of powerlessness. Nurses are not by nature 'political animals' and therefore are often not equipped to deal with essential political problems. Engineering an environment where nursing ethics and philosophies take precedence over institutional demands is a political activity and, as yet, nurses do not have the prerequisite skills to achieve this. The cause rests both with traditional approaches to management and the nurse's traditional approaches to nursing. They are both professionally and ethically juxtaposed, but one (by virtue of its control) renders the other subordinate and therefore relatively powerless. By doing so, its capacity for compromise is reduced, with the ultimate effect of reducing even more the creative power of the nurse and his or her clients. In effect, unless nurses act in a more positive and assertive fashion, this situation will not be resolved, to the detriment of nursing development.

NURSING ASSERTIVENESS

How can nurses assert themselves more effectively both within the clinical and political arenas? There are no simple answers, nor are they all ethical. From an ethical standpoint, the question should be rather: 'Should nurses assert themselves more?' When the qualities of assertive behaviour are considered, the sense of rightness that they produce, confidence, firmness, forcefulness, self-assurance and decisiveness, are not necessarily the features expected of a nurse involved in support, compromise and tolerant, caring behaviour. Unless nurses adopt some of these qualities, however, they lose credibility with both their managers and their clients. The main thrust of a nurse's endeavour should be to use these qualities in the appropriate way, and to best effect. 'Being assertive' is as skilled an activity as talking to bereaved persons, or counselling a child abuser, or being tolerant of those who manipulate others.

The nurse has to learn the skills of assertiveness in the same way as he or she had to learn the other relevant professional skills. Nurses have to learn how to promote themselves in different situations and with different people. Being assertive in a relationship with a client may mean sticking to a contract, and doing what has been agreed. Being assertive with a doctor may involve presenting a professional opinion about a client based upon scientific knowledge, precise and accurate clinical observations, and presenting the case for hearing the client's opinion and taking it into account in the decision-making process. Being assertive does not mean being dogmatic with the client, and pushy with the medical staff, to the point of becoming feared or disliked. The effects of assertiveness are to gain others' respect for forthrightness, and value from the role, or place in that setting. Being assertive enables the individual to develop his or her skills to produce a social climate of equality. Unfortunately many nurses do not assert themselves properly, or appropriately to the situation. Mrs Thatcher was more than assertive when Britain went to war with Argentina over the Falklands; such outright conflict and aggression within a clinical environment would be totally unacceptable. Assertiveness is effectiveness — doing the right thing, at the right time, and in the right way. The ability to be assertive stems from certainty and confidence in actions and beliefs, which are based upon knowledge and experience.

High stress, professional alienation, lack of peer support, inconclusive clinical results and lack of guidance have a detrimental effect on an individuals' confidence and their ability to be right (Ward, 1986). Ethically, a nurse cannot afford to be wrong; so how can a situation which produces such uncertainty be avoided?

The educational process should facilitate nursing assertiveness. Confidence in abilities comes from knowledge, not only of the subject, but abilities, beliefs and sense of purpose, knowledge of strengths and weaknesses which enables the person to use each in the most appropriate way, and to greatest effect. Self-awareness and self-expression form the basis of such understanding. If nurses are capable of such activities, they are more likely to promote them in their clients. Eventually client assertiveness, fostered by intuitive nurses, might resolve the problem of care emancipation, in which case the whole shape and style of care delivery will alter.

Educationalists however, can only take the nurse so far along the road of personal effectiveness. There should be a clear pattern of clinical support and supervision within the clinical area, with benign encouragement and reward for endeavour, as well as success. Most student nurses can recount horror stories of being left alone to cope with intolerable stress, difficult patients, overwhelming psychological pain and pure fear in situations where they should have been supported, counselled or simply *not* been left alone in the first place. It is not acceptable merely to say that all nurses have to go through these experiences, as this 'deep-end philosophy' is founded upon ignorance and a lack of caring. If nurses are to become really autonomous, self-reliant and purposeful, then they need to be shown how to behave. A child cannot expect to grow up successfully without effective role models; nurses need the same in their professional development.

One of the greatest of all leadership qualities is the ability to give responsibility to others, both as a confidence-booster, and as a reward. It may seem strange to talk of providing more work as a reward, but if a nurse feels that he or she is being trusted and viewed by others as capable and having worth, this is a reward that activates future growth and ulti- mately personal effectiveness. This does not, however, mean being left to deal with a client who requires intervention skills the nurse has not yet developed, then being criticized because the person becomes worse. In effect, it means the senior clinical staff should evaluate the current skills of the nurse, and identify potential for growth. Having done so, responsi- bility must be offered in line with capability, and increased as the nurse progresses. The nurse should be aware of what is on offer; just as in a 'patient-nurse' relationship, individuals need to know what is happening to them.

The results of such increases in nursing effectiveness should mean that nurses' advocacy skills on behalf of their clients are improved; they are more likely to allow people a greater share of care decisions if they feel confident enough in themselves not to worry about who makes the decisions as long as they are made. Clients are rewarded by enlightened nurses, who see the need for personal growth as a precondition for per- sonal effectiveness and adaptability. Ethically this reflects a normative approach to care-planning, as it demands of individuals the necessity to choose for themselves, and not have others choose for them. The consequences for non-assertive nurses within a care environment is that they simply will not have the confidence to let their clients have their own way.

ASSERTIVENESS AND COMMUNICATION

Psychiatric nursing is a discipline which revolves around communication. Without communication, modern psychiatric care would be reduced to the level of that available in the 18th century, where individuals were left to their own devices and allowed to experience depths of despair and anguish that few people could tolerate. There are many different types of communication. Within the assertiveness/communication equation, what is required is the ability of one individual to transmit to another a sense of tolerance, rather than a verbal message of intent. This is best achieved by actions and deeds, as opposed to spelling out what will happen.

Nurses can contrive situations where people are given responsibility, and allowed to express themselves, without being told they can do so, yet allowing the nurse to retain control over that situation. For example, if a person had low feelings of worth, voiced feeling of personal incompe- tence, was sad, lonely and dejected, then the nurse — by using knowledge of the person's previous strengths — could show insight into this person's feelings and present capabilities. This could be in an informal discussion, or a practical activity. Non-critical rewards (or simple empathy) could be offered for this realization, even if the conclusion were wrong, inappropriate or negative. The person would soon realize after several events that it was acceptable to say or do what was wanted, whilst the nurse was fully aware of the dynamics of the interactions. As the situation progressed, so the nurse would alter the pattern of the interaction, and begin to set tasks and objectives which could be rewarded, despite the person's ability (or inability) to achieve them successfully. This expressive, not objective, approach to the relationship would generate feelings of confidence, which might form the basis of a more positive personal development (i.e. give hope where there is none).

In this example, there is a clear danger of a manipulation in the guise of nursing care; this type of 'contingency management' would have to be framed in a contact between nurse and client. This, however, is just one example. How an individual nurse engineers a situation whereby his or her personal effectiveness enables another person to learn from his or her own mistakes is as personal and intimate as the relationship that exists between any one nurse and client. The ethical problem is not whether it should be done, nor even how it is done, but more importantly what happens. Such activities represent real control, or power. The ability of one individual to use his or her personal strengths to influence another person is a common theme throughout history. The nurse, however, should use this power so that the client may reclaim the position of an equal. This means (amongst other things) that nurses should also be aware of what they are doing, and pass that knowledge on to other members of their clinical team, so that they can either use that skill themselves within the working relationship, or simply maintain the continuity of the intervention within their own planning activities. Assertiveness is therefore about communicating strengths to another person, so that he or she feels confident enough, and safe enough to be wrong or expose their innermost feelings of weakness and failure, in the hope that by exploring these depths that learning will occur. Transmitting that strength is a skill that stems from confidence, whilst passing that information on to colleagues is an ethical obligation to clients.

WHY CHANGE?

Do nurses actually need to make changes in the ways they carry out their care planning activities? Is their ethical strategy strong enough to support (or even warrant) such notions? Do psychiatric clients want more effective nurses? Do other disciplines really want capable and autonomous nurses? The answer to all these questions must be a resounding, 'yes'. The reason is very simple. Nurses are probably closer to what is regarded as a helping agency than any other discipline within psychiatry. Their contact time sets them apart from all others. To have clients leave hospitals, clinics or 'community care' despite nurses (rather than because of them) would be a sad reflection on a profession whose main aim is to promote personal competence, satisfaction and achievement. A large shift in clinical intent is not required, simply a realization that professional assertiveness, linked with the human virtues inherent within a consequentialist sense of purpose, must be part of professional psychiatric nursing. Thinking of the client as an equal is a relatively modern concept. Certainly, as approaches to care planning are traced through recent psychiatric history, this sense of sharing has not been a common theme. Promoting client emancipation within a care environment and allowing those people to make supported mistakes without chastisement, will constitute an enormous alteration in the direction of normative ethics. Nursing professionalism will not emerge as a consequence of copying the behaviours of other disciplines, but by establishing true caring professionalism indicative of nurses.

CONCLUSIONS

To be able to project theories and hypotheses into the future is not only a difficult but also a risky activity. The need for change (and the desire to create an environment where care actually works) is probably a wish of many nurses. In psychiatry, where there are relatively low power differentials and interdisciplinary communication is quite good, there is certainly the right kind of atmosphere to allow such change to take place. Unfortunately, change has to be seen as necessary by those with the overall power to sanction change if it is to occur rapidly. In this situation, this is not the case. Establishing a nursing ethos based upon utilitarianism and consequentialistic theory is not just something that can be enforced, or written down or even taught, because it is about beliefs and attitudes. Nurses have to believe that their clients are their equals, if they are to use ethical theory to best advantage.

Care-planning, with all its inherent activities, is only truly effective if both the nurse and the client see it as being significant — and significance only occurs through participation. Nurses need to participate in their own professional developments, and become aware of the forces that motivate them as individuals. They need to allow their clients to develop and experience more than the contrived environment of 'parental' or 'policing' psychiatry. People have to be given the opportunity to be as assertive as their nurses, because it is their ultimate right to choose. Actions which they then carry out will be 'right' in proportion to their own need, and as a consequence promote happiness or satisfaction. Decisions made for them by others may well produce the reverse effects. Happiness is a feeling of pleasure and the absence of physical or psychological pain — lack of happiness, with its attendant privation of pleasure and satisfaction, is not the object of sound ethical approaches or good quality nursing intervention.

The ethical issues and difficulties discussed above are common to all psychiatric nurses. Debates about whether familiarity is harmful or constructive, whether patients should dictate care strategies, whether nurses should be more forthright, whether power and control interfere with a nurse's ability to carry out real human nursing, and debates on many other issues, will always take place. The need to establish an ethical approach to care planning for all nurses and their clients based upon mutual understanding, tolerance and personal confidence — normative ethics — remains paramount. Consequentialism, with its belief in human goodness and the struggle to achieve what is good in life forms an admirable backdrop for this approach. Ultimately, it is the quality of the nurse that determines the quality of the person, for an effective and confident nurse will facilitate the growth of an effective and confident client.

REFERENCES

Allen, H. (1981) Voices of concern: A study of verbal communications about patients in a psychiatric day unit. *Journal of Advanced Nursing* **6**, 355–362.

Brooking, J. I. (1988) A scale to measure use of nursing process. *Nursing Times*, **84** (15), 44–49.

Bottorff, J. L. and D'Cruz, J. V. (1984) Towards inclusive notions of 'patient' and 'nurse'. *Journal of Advanced Nursing*, **9** (15), 44–49.

Brown, P., Funsch, P. *et al.* (1987) Linking psychiatric nursing care to patient classification codes. *Nursing and Health Care*, **8** (3) 157–164.

Coler, M. S. and Vincent, K. G. (1987) Coded nursing diagnosis on Axis: A prioritized, computer ready, diagnostic system for psychiatric/ mental health nurses. *Archives of Psychiatric Nursing*, **1** (2), 125–131.

De la Cuesta, C. (1983) *Nursing Process. From Theory to Implementation*. Unpublished MSc thesis, University of London.

Ehrman, M. L. (1988) Using a factored patient classification system in psychiatry. *Nursing Management*, **18**, (5), 48–53.

Jameton, A. (1984) *Nursing Practice: The Ethical Issues*. Prentice Hall, Englewood Cliffs, N. J.

Jones, J. A. (1988) Clinical reasoning in nursing. *Journal of Advanced Nursing*, **13**, 185–192.

Keddy, B. (1985) The doctor-nurse relationship: an historical perspective. *Journal of Advanced Nursing*, **11**, 745–753.

Lebow, J. (1982) Consumer satisfaction with mental health treatment. *Psychological Bulletin*, **91**, (2), 244–259.

Morrison, P. (1989) Nursing and caring: a personal construct theory study of some nurses self perception. *Journal of Advanced Nursing*, **14**, 421–426.

Norris, J. and Kuens-Connell, M. (1988) A multimodel approach to validation and refinement of an existing nursing diagnosis. *Archives of Psychiatric Nursing*, **2**, (2), 103–109.

Raatikainen, R. (1989) Values and ethical principles in nursing. *Journal of Advanced Nursing*, **14**, 92–96.

Shields, P. J. (1985) The consumer view of psychiatry. *Hospital and Health Service Review*, **81**, 117–119.

Shields, P. J., Morrison, P. and Hart, D. (1988) Consumer satisfaction on a psychiatric ward. *Journal of Advanced Nursing*, **13**, 396–400.

Thiroux, J. P. (1980) *Ethics, Theory and Practice*, 2nd ed. Glencoe Publishing, Encino, C. A.

Topf, M. (1988) Verbal interpersonal responses. *Journal of Psychosocial Nursing*, **26** (7), 8–16.

Trusted, J. (1979) *The Logic of Scientific Interference*. Macmillan, London.

Tschudin, V (1986) *Ethics in Nursing: The Caring Relationship*. Heinemann, London.

UKCC (1984) *Code of Professional Conduct*. United Kingdom Central Council for Nurses, Midwives and Health Visitors, London.

van Maanen, H. M. (1984) Evaluation of care: A multinational perspective. In Willis, L. D. and Linwood, M. E. (eds.) *Measuring the Quality of Care*. Churchill Livingstone, Edinburgh.

Ward, M. F. (1985) *The Nursing Process in Psychiatry*, Churchill Livingstone, Edinburgh.

Ward, M. F. (1986) *Primary Nursing in Psychiatry: A Realistic Appraisal of Practice*. Nursing Process Link 9. ENB Learning Resources Unit, Sheffield.

Ward, M. F. (1988) The nursing process. In Kreb, M. J. and Larson, K. (eds.) *Applied Psychiatric/Mental Health Nursing Standards in Clinical Practice*. John Wiley, New York.

Chapter Nine

Ethics and clinical practice: a behavioural analysis

Chris Cullen

EDITORS' INTRODUCTION

What people 'do', rather than what they 'say' they do, represents the true heart of ethics. For those concerned to 'help' people with some handicap or disability, whether or not their actions 'work' is of paramount importance. A central debate exists about whether it is ethical to use techniques which realize objectives, whatever the cost, rather than use methods which are less effective, but less costly. This debate is of greatest relevance to people with major handicaps or disabilities: the groups who, traditionally, have had the least influence over the kind of services they receive. The selection of 'appropriate' interventions, by professionals, is most often determined by peer group pressure, rather than by a rational assessment of outcome.

This assumes that the selection, and ultimate assessment of the effectiveness of different interventions is a one-way process: that recipients have no part to play. Whether or not professionals act upon service recipients in this manner is open to question. In this chapter **Chris Cullen** presents an analysis of control in therapy: what actually causes or determines 'change'. This question is vital to both the setting of treatment goals and the selection of methods deemed to be appropriate, or necessary, to realize those aims.

Ethics and clinical practice: a behavioural analysis

The study of ethics had been the mainstay of philosophers for many years. They have argued and debated the relation between 'is' and 'ought', and how this might (or might not) be relevant to everyday life. Such debates, however, have had very little impact for most people. As Karl Marx observed: 'The philosophers have only interpreted the world in various ways; the point however is to change it'.

When people talk about what they do, or ought to do, they are talking about behaviour. Technically, it is verbal behaviour determined (brought about or influenced) by other social behaviour (see for example Skinner, 1957), although the fine detail of a behavioural analysis is not relevant here. It seems reasonable to assume, therefore, that a behaviourist perspective can add something useful to the debate. In particular, some of the ways in which a behaviourist approach identifies the determinants of everyday professional lives in clinical practice will be examined.

BEHAVIOURISM AND ETHICS

Behaviourists have contributed to the philosophical debate, as well as to more practical issues. Some of the most exciting examples of the former are to be found in the various writings of B. F. Skinner (1978, 1987). Although widely misunderstood (Wheeler, 1973) behaviourism has been described as: '. . . an important work of moral philosophy, possibly the most important produced in our time' (Hocutt, 1977). It is a thoroughgoing analysis of many of the concepts traditionally taken to be the domain of moral philosophers, and has led to radical behaviourism becoming almost a household name.

That contribution of behaviourism, however, is more concerned with the wider issues of the nature of society and is not the focus of this chapter. A behavioural analysis can help cast light on the day-to-day therapeutic practices of the helping professions, in particular via decision-making in therapy (Stolz, 1978). The various behaviours which make up the complex repertoire referred to as 'therapeutic behaviour', have been a particularly important and practical contribution.

CONTROL AND COUNTER-CONTROL

Central to the philosophy of radical behaviourism is the notion that all behaviour is determined. It is part of a physical system and, potentially at least, the determinants of behaviour can be identified. If the causes of behaviour are known there is some possibility of prediction and control, and this is the aim of a science of behaviour (Hayes and Brownstein, 1986). Unfortunately, the term 'control', (although used by behaviourists in the same sense as 'determine' or 'cause') has been taken by non-behaviourists to imply threats to human dignity.

If all behaviour is determined or controlled, then it follows that the behaviour of those in positions of power or authority (such as teachers, judges and therapists) must be determined by something. Influences on their behaviour are the substance of this chapter. The extent to which their behaviour is determined by the behaviour of those over whom they have authority has been termed **counter-control** (Skinner, 1974). The behaviour of person A is influenced in a significant way by the behaviour of person B, and person B also exerts some influence over the behaviour of person A: control and counter-control. The balance may be equal or unequal, depending on the situation. The prisoner-jailer relation is generally more unequal than the wife-husband relation.

In therapy, it is usually assumed that the balance is relatively unequal. An extreme case is quoted:

> I believe, as a physician who has prior contact with the family, that I can persuade 99 percent of my patients to my way of thinking if I really work at it, even if I am 100 percent wrong. If I tell them in such a way that I appear concerned and that I am knowledgeable and that I have their interest at heart and the interest of their fetus or their new-born baby, there is no question in my mind but that they will let me 'cut off the infant's head'.
>
> (Goldiamond, 1974)

Therapists seem to have more power over their clients than do clients over therapists. This unequal balance of power has led society to devise external means, on behalf of the recipients of therapy, of counter-controlling the behaviour of therapists (i.e. of ensuring that therapists' main concerns are the welfare of their clients). Stolz (1978) has reviewed various laws and guidelines promulgated by national and international bodies which regulate therapeutic practice; without exception, what they all have in common is attention to obvious contingencies of control, such as extortion by therapists, deliberate harming, and taking advantage of clients.

The control of behaviour is sometimes very subtle, however:

> A whip is a more obvious instrument of control than wages, and wages are more conspicuous than sacerdotal privileges, and privileges are more obvious than the prospect of an affluent future life . . . We are likely to single out the conspicuous example of control, because in their abruptness and clarity of effect, they seem to start something, but it is a great mistake to ignore the inconspicuous forms.
>
> (Skinner, 1971)

For clinical practice, Stolz (1978) argued that the more subtle forms of control are very important and need to be understood. In general, society can legislate to prevent conspicuous abuse of power, but inconspicuous abuse is much harder to deal with. It has often been argued that only by making sources of control clear, will people be able to work towards a better world (Skinner, 1948). If there already exist ways of counter-controlling the effects of lust and greed — although there is plenty of room to doubt the effectiveness of such procedures — some of the subtle and inconspicuous factors which might determine therapists' behaviour should be considered.

CONTROL IN THERAPY

Stolz (1978) identified seven components which were referred to as the stages of decision-making in therapy. They were:

1. identifying the client;
2. deciding if an intervention is necessary;
3. selecting goals;
4. choosing an intervention strategy;
5. obtaining informed consent;
6. preparing a description of alternative goals and means; and
7. making decisions about goals and means.

From a behaviourist viewpoint, the crucial issue is that the terms emphasized in each stage are terms which describe or refer to behaviour. These behaviours are susceptible to many determinants: some conspicuous, and some subtle. For example, a client might report sexual fantasies about young children which resulted in unbearable feelings of guilt. The strong social control over the behaviour of the therapist might immediately advise an intervention aimed at suppressing paedophiliac, and increasing adult, sexual behaviour.

The possible contingencies of control in just one of the stages of therapy — choosing an intervention — will be examined. This is not the result of an extensive survey of sources of control amongst different therapists, nor an attempt to manipulate an environment to demonstrate that the inferred sources of control are actually operating as an essential step in a functional analysis (Cullen 1983). Rather they are some guesses based on less-than systematic observations of personal behaviour, and that of close colleagues. The account is intended to be no more than illustrative. Although accounts of functional analyses of behaviour should be consistent, these descriptions will not be adequately technological (Baer, *et al.*, 1987) and will sometimes be 'mentalistic' (Moore, 1981). It is occasionally helpful, however, to be interpretative, and at least it serves the function of raising awareness of likely determinants of behaviour.

SOME DETERMINANTS OF THE CHOICE OF A THERAPEUTIC INTERVENTION

In an ideal world, therapists would always do whatever was 'best' for their clients, and no other consideration would enter the equation. That is probably how most clients see their therapist, or physician, when illness strikes. Unfortunately, this is not an ideal world, and often there is little consensus on what is best for the client. Accordingly, advice given to the same client with the same set of problems can vary widely from therapist to therapist. A personal anecdote clearly illustrates this:

In 1987 I was one of a group intending to climb a mountain. It is well known that climbers who ascend too rapidly often have altitude sickness, comprising headaches and nausea. High altitude mountaineers are aware that acetazolamide is good at preventing altitude sickness, although there is the risk that by so doing it might mask the symptoms of pulmonary or, more seriously, cerebral oedema, both of which if not quickly treated can result in death. Furthermore, acetazolamide is not manufactured for use in high altitude mountaineering. My own physician refused to prescribe the drug for me; my friend's physician prescribed the drug without question. Clearly my physician was taking into account factors such as his own professional liability, and my longer-term interests, whereas my friend's physician was more influenced by the shorter-term problems of altitude sickness we were about to face. I doubt that either doctor stopped to do more than a cursory analysis of the determinants of their behaviour.

Some advice will benefit the client more than other advice, but most practising clinicians are not aware of anything more than the most dominant influences on their therapeutic behaviour. So what are the possibilities?

Client behaviour

Hopefully, predicted and actual improvement in the client will be a major determinant of therapist behaviour. Anything which results in deterioration should not occur. Therapy should be devised leading to the quickest and/or most permanent positive changes. This implies that day-to-day clinical practice should be experimental in nature, with the therapist regularly manipulating conditions and using appropriate research designs to evaluate effects. Clinicians should constantly explore new combinations of variables, monitor change, and reject the least beneficial. The constructional approach (Schwartz and Goldiamond, 1975) provides an excellent example of such an approach.

This is not necessarily the practice of most therapists however. Those therapists who do seem to be operating in this fashion, as reported in journals or at conferences, sound marvellous and it can lead to despair for others.

There are many other aspects of the client's repertoire which might determine therapist behaviour. For example, it would be interesting to monitor the amount of time given by therapists to young, attractive clients compared with that given to dirty, depressed and deformed clients. In the context of the British NHS (where clients pay nothing directly to therapists) the control of clinician's behaviour by the fee paid by clients is difficult to appreciate, but this can also be a particular potent influence. In their witty and iconoclastic examination of how to be a successful psychotherapist, no matter what the effect on behaviour, Epling and Woodward (1976) identified one of the major canons of psychotherapy as: 'the therapist must continue to be paid, regularly and lavishly'.

Facilities

The physical work settings of clinicians may play a significant part in determining the therapy they offer. For example, if a residence for people with a mental handicap has a safe and secure room specifically designed for time-out procedures, then there is a good chance it will be used. It may also be used for a variety of purposes, other than properly constituted time-out procedures, including simply removing the handicapped person to reduce annoyance to staff regardless of the longer-term effect on that person's behaviour. In places without such facilities, time-out will be unlikely to figure out the therapies on offer, and other procedures to deal with challenging behaviour will emerge.

A common current practice is the use of various kinds of relaxation training and biofeedback. To offer such therapies, clinicians have to purchase expensive equipment, such as reclining chairs and physiological monitoring devices. The literature on the effectiveness of such interventions, however, suggest little cause for optimism. Differential effects achieved with relaxation techniques and biofeedback have not yet been shown to have tremendous clinical importance, and certainly not when used in isolation from a programme aimed at increasing clients' behavioural repertoires. The equipment purchase however seems to set the occasion for its use.

Fashion

'What everyone else is doing' undoubtedly influences the behaviour of most therapists. Some years ago it was fashionable to be a 'behaviour modifier', and many therapists described themselves thus, or at least had behaviour modification as one of their armoury of techniques. That term lost its value for various reasons and was replaced by 'functional analysis'. Clinicians who describe their versions of 'functional analysis' could lead to a belief that few know much about the term, its genesis, or how one might go about doing it (Cullen, 1983). More recently, the term 'constructional approach' has been used to describe essentially the same therapies which used to be described as 'behaviour modification'. The constructional approach, which is a specific type of therapy, was devised by Israel Goldiamond (Goldiamond, 1974; Schwartz and Goldiamond, 1975) but a recent text with the term in its title (Zarkowska and Clements, 1988) does not even mention the basic tenets as set out by Goldiamond and his colleagues.

Since 1980, many clinicians have turned to 'cognitive therapy'. Colleagues who have adopted this approach state that it is because of the failure of behaviourism to deal with the feelings and emotions of their clients. This was the message of Mahoney (1974) in his writings on cognition and behaviour modification. A critical examination of Mahoney's arguments reveals, however, that there is very little to concern the radical behaviourist (Cullen and Gathercole, 1976; Rachlin, 1977). Mahoney (and other cognitive therapists) either have not understood, or have misrepresented or failed to address, the radical behaviourist position.

It is strange that the cognitive fashion should have taken hold. The foundations of cognitive therapy, and the data on which it is apparently based, are somewhat precarious (Cullen, 1980). As long ago as 1974, Mahoney was forced to conclude of one of bases of the cognitive approach that: 'the empirical evidence on the effectiveness of procedures derived from the covert conditioning model tentatively suggest that its clinical utility may be problem-specific and summarily modest' (Mahoney, 1974).

Little has happened in the cognitive therapy field in the intervening years to allow a challenge of that conclusion. A recent study examining the outcomes of different types of therapy favoured prescriptive therapies over exploratory therapies, although they had curiously described the prescriptive therapies as 'cognitive/behavioural' (Shapiro and Firth, 1987).

Avoidance of disapproval

Sometimes, therapy which is effective for the client may be rather like the discomfort experienced by visits to the dentist; short-term pain for long-term benefit. Usually therapists have little trouble in handing out nasty medicine to their clients; they may for example advise a parent to ignore the tantrums of a difficult child. In the short-term things will get worse, but in the long-term benefit will be worth the trouble.

Occasionally, however, the short-term discomfort is experienced by the therapist, as well as by the client, and may come from society in general, or from professional peers. A good example is the avoidance of punishment procedures by many clinicians when dealing with severe self-injurious behaviour. When faced with particularly strong self-destructive behaviour in people with a mental handicap, it may be necessary to consider the use of punishment procedures. That therapists rarely do so in practice is almost certainly associated with the disapproval of colleagues, and society in general. A poignant scenario is given:

> A colleague at a different university showed us a deeply moving film. The heroine was an institutionalized primary-grade girl. She was a headbanger, so a padded football helmet was put on her head. Because she could take it off, her hands were tied down in her crib. She kept tossing her neck and tore out her hair at every opportunity. She accordingly had a perpetually bruised face on a hairless head, with neck almost as thick as that of a horse. She was nonverbal.
>
> My colleague and his staff carefully planned a program for her, using

all kinds of reinforcers. She was remanded to their program, but persisted in her typical behaviour. In desperation, the ultimate weapon was unwrapped. When she tossed her head, my colleague yelled 'Don't', simultaneously delivering a sharp slap to her cheek. She subsided for a brief period, tossed again, and the punishment was delivered. My colleague reports that less than a dozen slaps were ever delivered and that the word 'Don't!' yelled even from across the room was effective. Its use was shortened down to once a week and was discontinued in a few weeks. In the meantime, the football helmet was removed and the girl began to eat at the table. She slept in a regular bed. Her hair grew out, and she turned out to be a very pretty little blond girl with delicate features and a delicate neck. In less than a year, she started to move towards joining a group of older girls whose behaviour, it was hoped, she would model. She smiled often.

The initial institution and her parents discovered that she had been slapped. They immediately withdrew her from the custody of my colleague's staff. The last part of the film shows her back at the institution. She is strapped down in her crib. Her hands are tied to her sides. She is wearing a football helmet. Her hair is torn out, her face a mass of bruises and her neck is almost as thick as that of a horse.

(Goldiamond, 1974)

The use of aversive contingencies in cases of self-destructive behaviour is not condoned. The use of mild aversive electrical stimulation for people with mental handicaps who give themselves self-injurious blows to the head via a device (SIBIS, developed by Human Technologies, Inc.) has provided a major controversy in the United States of America. Many practitioners have eschewed the use of aversive (in favour of non-aversive) procedures, even where there is limited data to support the available non-aversive procedures (Axelrod, 1987) and some support for the effectiveness of some punishment procedures (e.g. Jordan *et al.*, 1989). Some therapists have opposed the use of aversive/punishing procedures for fear of 'what colleagues will say', rather than on a discerning examination of the literature, or a careful conceptual analysis (Sidman, 1989).

Immediate reinforcement and least effort

Some therapeutic practice is undoubtedly determined by the immediate effect a client can have on therapist behaviour. A clear, simple example is deciding where to meet the client. It is easiest, but more inconvenient for the client, to make appointments for meetings at the therapist's office, or in the department clinic. It is much more convenient for clients to be visited in their own home, preferably in the evening. This is however maximally inconvenient for the therapist. There is little evidence to indicate that appointments in one setting are better for client improvement, than appointments in another. Therapists rationalize that they can see more people, and that clients are more likely to be motivated to change, if they have clinics. They could also argue however, that advice will be based on a more full knowledge of the clients' lifestyle and circumstances if they are visited in their own home.

So, some therapists make a point of visiting clients in their own home. Clients are pleased and grateful, and colleagues are impressed at devotion above and beyond the call of duty. For some professionals, there is also the additional factor of a financial incentive, for visiting clients at home or out of normal hours.

There is also the obverse. Some therapists may see clients in clinics or offices because it is easier. Parents and young children often visit child guidance clinics; the 'terrible child' is sitting reading, or playing quietly. The parent is worried that the psychologist will not be able to understand that the child never sits quietly at home. In such cases, it might be much better for the psychologist to see the contingencies in effect at home, since the parent's description of them is very likely to be inaccurate or inadequate. However, the 'principle of least effort' can be very powerful in determining behaviour.

Social contingencies

Holland (1978), argued that behaviourism may be seen as part of the problem, as well as part of the solution, and pointed out that aversive procedures are used when clients have behaviours which society regards as dangerous or unpleasant — behaviour such as alcohol abuse and sexual offences. Somehow it then seems reasonable to arrange contingencies which lead to an alcohol abuser becoming violently sick, or using electric shock as a punisher with a sex offender. Although it might be as effective, it would be unacceptable to shock a person who had sought help for shyness whenever he or she averted the gaze. Holland's analysis is compelling — often there seems to be a sense in which 'the therapy fits the problem'.

Therapist history and training

The effect of training and history should not be overlooked; it is likely to be all-pervasive. If the 'ultimate' study were to be published (demonstrating the superiority of behavioural therapies over psychotherapies) it would have little effect on the clinical behaviour of psychotherapists. The reasons are obvious. Once a long and intensive training has been undertaken, and a new, unique and complex verbal and clinical repertoire has been established, it will take more than 'benefits to clients' to change things. Major shifts in orientation — in any field of human endeavour — are sufficiently rare for them to be noteworthy (Kuhn, 1962).

In the field of mental handicap, normalization (Wolfensberger, 1972) or social role valorization (Wolfensberger, 1983) is the current watchword. This defined as:

> Utilization of means which are as culturally normative as possible, in order to establish, enable, or support behaviour, appearances and interpretations which are as culturally normative as possible.
>
> (Wolfenberger, 1972)

To assess the degree of conformity to the normalization principle, Wolfensberger and his colleagues have developed an evaluation system known as PASS (Wolfensberger and Glenn, 1975). Before a full operation is possible of the implications of normalization for service delivery, (and before using PASS) an intensive training is needed. This often takes the form of a week-long workshop, during which participants are given what comes close to a religious conversion experience. Needless to say, many of those who undergo the experience become avid proponents of PASS and the normalization principle: such proselytizing has been criticized (Baldwin, 1985).

Whilst many people are sympathetic to the principle of normalization — because they share a common history and culture with its proponents — many people are puzzled by the lack of empirical evidence on which some of its canons are based. For example, what is the optimal size for living units? In what way is a living unit of six people always better than one of twenty? Staff behaviour is unrelated to size of the facility, and residents of larger facilities may be engaged in more social behaviour than those in smaller facilities (Landesman-Dwyer *et al.*, 1980). This sort of study may give research a 'bad name'. Therapist history and training may also be capable of working against the best interests of clients.

The determinants of therapist behaviour discussed above are easily overlooked. They are interrelated, and the list is not exhaustive. There are other contingencies in therapy which may seem simple, but which (on closer examination) turn out to be complex. The token economies set up in large institutions in the late 1960s are one example. They were introduced because of obvious benefits to clients and, it was argued, such a system was more 'humane' because it allowed previously devalued people to manipulate and arrange their own environments. The token economy system appeared to be benign, and the very antithesis of extant regimes were clearly coercive.

Turning the analytical system of behaviourism onto some technologies (the token economy for example) has demonstrated that they are maximally coercive rather than benign (Goldiamond, 1974, 1975, 1976). Goldiamond's analysis of ethical behaviour, and of coercion in particular, is complex. The essence of the analysis, however, is that both the obvious contingencies, and the alternatives, should be considered. For example, in a **negative reinforcement** procedure:

1. Ongoing program participation leads to a decrease in aversive density;
2. Not participating in the programme leads to maintenance of aversive density.

One example might be where 'agreeing' to take part in medical research in a prison is rewarded with privileges, or early release. It is only when non-participation is considered that the coercive nature of the paradigm becomes clear.

In a **positive reinforcement** paradigm, (such as the typical token economy) reinforcement is made contingent on only one behaviour. Any alternative behaviour leads to the withholding of reinforcement — this is clearly coercive.

There are two common ways in which systems set up such coercion. The first is institutionally instigated, where the system first deprives people of certain goods or privileges, and then allows them to earn them back. The second is institutionally opportune, where the system takes advantages of opportunities which it has not specifically created. An example of the latter is when medical treatment is available only on payment of a fee.

These coercive scenarios are interrelated, and may operate together in many so-called therapeutic situations. One of the grossest examples has been reported by Cotter (1967). In a Vietnamese mental hospital, patients were: firstly, told they could go home if they worked first for a period of three months; secondly, given electro-convulsive therapy if they still refused to work; and thirdly, deprived of food if they did not work (working was reinforced with food). Other no less unsophisticated 'treatments' were also described.

CONCLUSIONS

Because behaviourism addresses the issue of how and why people do things, and addresses the issue of ways which can lead to prediction and control, it is particularly suited to an analysis of ethics. Behaviourists contribute to the academic/philosophical debate, and also the question of control of therapists and others in positions of power. Unless behaviourists analyse and point out the controlling contingencies, then their value in society will not be fully realized.

REFERENCES

Axelrod, S. (1987) Doing it without arrows: a review of Lavigna and Donnellan's Alternatives to punishment: solving behaviour problems with non-aversive strategies. *The Behaviour Analyst*, **10**, 243–251.
Baer, D. M., Wolf, M.M. and Risley, T. R. (1987) Some still-current dimensions of applied behaviour analysis. *Journal of Applied Behaviour Analysis*, **20**, 313–327.
Baldwin, S. (1985) Sheep in wolf's clothing: Impact of normalization teaching on

human services and service providers. *International Journal of Rehabilitation Research*, **8**, 131–142.

Cotter, L. H. (1967) Operant conditioning in a Vietnamese mental hospital. *American Journal of Psychiatry*, **124**, 23–28.

Cullen, C. (1980) Questioning the foundations of cognitive behaviour modification. In Main, C. J. (ed.) *Clinical Psychology and Medicine: A Behavioural Perspective*. Plenum, New York.

Cullen, C. (1983) Implications of functional analysis. *British Journal of Clinical Psychology*, **22**, 137–138.

Cullen, C. and Gathercole, C. E. (1976) Review of Cognition and Behaviour Modification by M. J. Mahoney. *Bulletin of the British Association for Behavioural Psychotherapy*, **4**, 12–17.

Epling. W.F. and Woodward, J. B. (1976) How to be a successful psychotherapist no matter what the effect on behavior: The corn soup principle. *Behavior Research and Therapy*, **14**, 482–484.

Goldiamond, I. (1974) Towards a constructional approach to social problems. Ethical and constitutional problems raised by applied behavior analysis. *Behaviorism*, **2**, 1–84.

Goldiamond, I. (1975) Alternative sets as a framework for behavioral formulations and research. *Behaviorism*, **3**, 49–86.

Goldiamond, I. (1976) Protection of human subjects and patients. A social contingency analysis of distinction between research and practice and its implications. *Behaviourism*, **4**, 1–41.

Hayes, S. C. and Brownstein, A. J. (1986) Mentalism, behaviour — behaviour relations, and a behaviour — analytic view of the purposes of science, *The Behavior Analyst*, **9**, 175–190.

Hocutt, M. (1977) Skinner on the word 'good': a naturalistic semantics for ethics. *Ethics*, **87**, 319–338.

Holland, J. G. (1978) Behaviorism: part of the problem or part of the solution? *Journal of Applied Behaviour Analysis*, **11**, 163–174.

Jordan, J., Singh, N. N. and Repp, A. C. (1989) An evaluation of gentle teaching and visual screening in the reduction of stereotypy. *Journal of Applied Behavior Analysis*, **22**, 9–22.

Kuhn, T. S. (1962) *The Structure of Scientific Revolutions*. Chicago University Press, Chicago.

Landesman-Dwyer, S., Sackett, G. P and Kleinman, J. S. (1980) Relationship of size to resident and staff behavior in small community residences. *American Journal of Mental Deficiency*, **85**, 6–17.

Mahoney, M. J. (1974) *Cognition and Behaviour Modification*. Ballinger, Cambridge, Mass.

Moore, J. (1981) On mentalism, methodological behaviourism and radical behaviorism. *Behaviourism*, **9**, 55–77.

Rachlin, H. A. (1977) A review of M. J. Mahoney's Cogniton and Behaviour Modification. *Journal of Applied Behaviour Analysis*, **10**, 369–374.

Schwartz, A. and Goldiamond, I. (1975) *Social Casework: a Behavioral Approach*. Columbia University Press, New York.

Shapiro, D. A. and Firth, J. (1987) Prescriptive v exploratory psychotherapy: outcomes of the Sheffield psychotherapy project. *British Journal of Psychiatry*, **151**, 790–799.

Sidman, M. (1989) *Coercion and its Fallout*. Authors Cooperation Inc, Boston.

Skinner, B. F. (1948) *Walden II*. Macmillan Publishing Inc., New York.

Skinner, B. F. (1957) *Verbal Behavior*. Appleton Century Crofts, New York.

Skinner, B. F. (1971) *Beyond Freedom and Dignity*. Jonathan Cape, London.
Skinner, B. F. (1974) *About Behaviorism*. Jonathan Cape, London.
Skinner, B. F. (1978) *Reflection on Behaviourism and Society*. Prentice Hall, Englewood Cliffs, N. J.
Skinner, B. F. (1987) *Upon Further Reflection*. Prentice Hall, Englewood Cliffs, N.J.
Stolz, S. B. (1978) Ethics of social and educational interventions: Historical context and a behavioral analysis. In Catania, A. C. and Brigham, T. A. (eds.) *Handbook of Applied Behaviour Analysis, Social and Instructional Processes*. Irvington Publishers, New York.
Wheeler, H. (1973). *Beyond the Punitive Society*. Wildwood House, London.
Wolfensberger, W. (1972) *The Principle of Normalization in Human Services*. National Institute on Mental Retardation, Toronto.
Wolfensberger, W. (1983) Social role valorization: a proposed new term for the principle of normalization. *Mental Retardation*, **21**, 234–239.
Wolfensberger, W. and Glenn, L. (1975) *Program Analysis of Service Systems*, 3rd ed. National Institute on Mental Retardation, Toronto.
Zarkowska, E. and Clements, J. (1988) *Problem Behaviour in People with Severe Learning Disabilities: A Pratical Guide to a Constructional Approach*. Croom Helm, London.

Chapter Ten

Change not adjustment: the ethics of psychotherapy

PHIL BARKER AND STEVE BALDWIN

EDITORS' INTRODUCTION

Where people permit professionals to exercise influence upon them, it is often assumed that no serious ethical dilemmas exist. The traditional assumption that ethical dilemmas involve only interventions capable of causing physical harm needs to be challenged. All forms of psychosocial 'treatment' involve the exercise of some form of influence over people who are vulnerable, if only by virtue of their problems. This psychological vulnerability suggests that the distinction between 'treatments' with physical outcomes, and all others should be abandoned.

Although psychotherapy is often assumed to be a single concept, the means by which people are offered psychological help are multiple. If psychotherapy addresses 'problems of living', as some writers would suggest, the optional solutions are infinite. Assuming the uncertain status of 'psychotherapy' can a core set of ethical criteria be established? If all psychotherapy address problems of living, do all forms of help with problems of living qualify as psychotherapies?

Attention has been focused on 'psychotherapy' since this form of treatment (if indeed it is a form or treatment) is most typical of mental health services. Given that all mental health professionals are involved in a relationship with a vulnerable human being, the issues raised here are of universal relevance.

The ethics of psychotherapy

Ethical issues in mental health service delivery tend to revolve around invasive interventions: concerns regarding the side effects of physical psychiatric treatments, such as drug therapy or ECT; or the final outcome of invasion of the 'politics of the person', as in institutionalization or stigmatization through diagnosis. Contemporary mental health services still retain these traditional, perhaps essential, invasive elements, supported by a range of 'psychosocial interventions'. The therapeutic aims of traditional, invasive treatments are human, if not necessarily humanistic. They are used to relieve a hypothetical mental illness: to minimize distress or risk of danger to self or others. Despite the apparent virtue of such aims the therapeutic process has been challenged. Critics view the machinery of treatment as little more than a technical conspiracy against the person (Szasz, 1962), perhaps for the simple reason that such 'technical' interventions are manifestly visible: a sitting target for the armchair critic.

Although the aims of psychosocial interventions are similar to invasive methods (attempting to address and resolve personal and 'life' problems), their processes are, by contrast, 'non-invasive'. It might be assumed therefore, that 'the psychotherapies' present few ethical dilemmas. It should be pointed out that the term 'psychotherapy' is used here to refer to any formal interpersonal encounter or negotiation between 'therapist' and 'patient', individually or in groups, described as a 'therapeutic relationship'. As many as 250 such 'psychotherapies' have been identified (Herink, 1980). Traditional psychiatric treatments such as hospitalization and diagnosis might be seen as coercive and restrictive, drug therapy as inhibitory, and ECT as potentially damaging. But are less invasive interventions, such as psychotherapy, any less fraught with ethical dilemmas? Are all psychotherapies benign? Can the person in therapy suffer, even when involved as an integral part of the psychotherapeutic process?

THE CONTEXT OF PSYCHOTHERAPY

The need for psychotherapy arises, at least in part, from the manifold assumptions of our culture as to the 'meaning of life'. Society expects, as Smail (1978) astutely observed, that people should be happy, must be competent to reach the goals determined by their social position, must get on with others, should be sexually adjusted and should enjoy sex. Moreover, people should live in harmonious families, should find out what is their 'full potential' and should realize this potential. Given that people cannot, by and large, help being the way they are, they need an expert 'helper' to guide them away from the pathological psyche described by Freud and his followers, or towards the 'full humanness' described by Maslow: they need a psychotherapist.

Whatever else psychotherapists claim to do, an alien visitor might interpret their practice as involving some kind of mind-healing. Although psychotherapy, in its many forms, is practised more now by non-medical agencies, 'therapy', of all sorts, has it origins in medical healing (*therapeutae* is synonomous in Greek for *essaioi*, 'doctors'; *therapeutike*, [the art of] healing). In Szasz's (1978) view conventional (*sic*) therapy is less a 'healing' process, more one of social action, comprising a series of 'religious, rhetorical and repressive acts.' Much of Szasz's concern was based upon the covert nature of psychotherapy: the surface appearance disguising a process which rarely matched the description of what was 'said' to be done. The language of psychotherapy, in common with all language, is a powerful tool: as such it can be used to control, as well as to describe people. Do recipients of the various therapies expect that their psyches will be healed? Do therapists wittingly deceive those they purport to 'treat'? How far has psychotherapy progressed from its original affinity with magic (Thomas, 1973; Karle, 1989)?

This chapter considers the act of psychotherapy from this semantic perspective: what do 'psychotherapists' say are the problems of the person whom they aim to help, and what do they say they do in the name of one therapy or another? The potential discrepancy between what is stated and what is, ultimately, enacted in 'therapy' is acknowledged: this may represent a further ethical dilemma for the practitioner of psychosocial intervention, but is beyond the scope of this chapter.

THE SCIENCE OF PSYCHOTHERAPY

Consideration of ethical issues in the practice of psychotherapy begins with the apparent conflict between psychotherapy (a presumed science) and ethics (a moral code). The following argument will suggest that psychotherapy, of whatever persuasion, is no more than a special body of knowledge which assumes a privileged status: in particular, freedom from the obligation to submit to the conventions of traditional sciences (see for example, Edelson, 1977).

Science might be defined as the reality that has been 'discovered': ethics involves recommendations, wishes, desires and prescriptions, for how the world should be. The psychotherapist helps people to move towards some adjusted, improved or ideal state: ambitions which are founded solidly upon human values which are largely moral in character. This aim appears to be common to most psychotherapies, although the methods used to pursue this differ. Some psychotherapies are involved with hermeneutics: purporting to probe beneath the surface significance of human action, seeking a more profound understanding of the person. Some allow the 'patient' to determine the exact nature of the change desired or needed. Such 'goal-setting' reflects a further moral dimension, or philosophy, with little in common with the world of science. Although much effort has been made to try to evaluate the 'art' of psychotherapy using scientific methods, the ethical location of psychotherapy may lie somewhere between the ideological extremes of an objectively applied science, and a code of healthy conduct (Erickson, 1976).

ROOTS AND BRANCHES

It is commonly assumed that the origins, or aetiology of a disorder must be uncovered before any significant treatment can be applied. This misconception is founded in a crude translation of the medical model of physical illness, unfitted to the problems of living described as 'mental disorders'. Davison and Neale (1986) note that the assumption that: 'a determinant of behaviour that is assumed to lie in the unconscious or past is somehow more 'underlying' or 'basic' than a determinant that is anchored in the current environment (p. 522)' is no more than an assumption'. They argue further that: 'if "underlying" is defined as "not immediately obvious", [even] behaviour therapists search for underlying causes (p.522)'. It should not be forgotten that the successful medical treatment of many physical disorders, such as diabetes or hypertension, is possible without addressing directly the 'historical cause' of the illness: assuming that control of the disorder is seen as 'successful' treatment. Despite these arguments, psychotherapeutic methods which do not address the historical (underlying) antecedents, such as behavioural or cognitive therapies, are considered no more than 'symptomatic'. At one level, these theoretical differences reflect no more than ideological conflicts. The base material seems to be identical across all therapies: psychotherapy 'is a situation in which one human being (the therapist) tries to act in such a way as to enable another human being to act and feel differently' (Wachtel, 1977).

The idea that the *proper* explanation of current psychological problems lies in suppressed memories of past experiences is one view of the genesis of 'psychopathology'. This crude characterization of psychoanalytic thought suggests that there is only one true, or proper, explanation and that such truth 'exists', rather than is constructed by the individual, in the form of some personal belief system; or by society, in the form of a consensus view. The idea that truth is 'made', rather than 'found' is a relatively new idea: Rorty (1989) observed that at least in Europe, the idea was less than 200 years old, being contemporaneous with the French Revolution. Utopian politics, as Rorty acknowledged, displaced notions concerning the will of God and the fundamental nature of Man (*sic*), resulting in the idea that society created 'man' or even that Man (*sic*) created himself. This issue is no mere academic trifle. The search for an acceptable model of the genesis and 'treatment' of problems of living generates the question: 'do such problems arise "within" the person, or are they a function of the person's relationship with him/herself in particular, and the world in general?' (Szasz, 1962).

THEORIES OF THERAPY

Despite the wide range of therapeutic possibilities, the likely offerings, even in the most sufficient of treatment settings, would cover no more than the following: psychodynamic psychotherapy (developed from Freud's original formulations); behavioural psychotherapy (derived from the application of various learning theories); and various 'humanistic' therapies. Such distinctions are theoretical or, in the absence of any testable theory, ideological in nature. In ethical terms it may be more appropriate to distinguish therapies by their arms, and the expectations (perhaps implicit) of the person in therapy. A distinction can be made between therapies which might be called 'traditional', humanistic or transpersonal (Banet, 1976). Using this approach, therapies can be distinguished by their view of the 'person', his or her motivation, assumed personal and social goals, as well as the process and practical focus of the therapy.

Traditional therapies such as psychoanalysis, its many psychodynamic derivatives, and the behavioural and cognitive therapies, share many of the features of hospitalization and physical forms of psychiatric treatment. Their assumptions include the idea of a mental life (or self) which owes most to Freud's ego psychology, itself no more than a translation of traditional Western cultural concepts of 'the person'. Even therapies which reject Freudian theory, such as behaviour therapy, replace it with similar 'mechanistic' and reductionist models of the person, who is defined primarily by others. The concept of 'normality' is central: emotional, intellectual and behavioural 'facets' of the person are described in terms of his or her position on a scale of normal functioning. The motivation for therapy is assumed to be a 'need' for change: on a personal level this means adjustment (the person is 'maladjusted') and on a broader social plane, increased socialization. The therapeutic process is assumed to involve 'ego building' or, more generally, healing. Behavioural approaches might deny that the person is 'sick' and in need of healing, but would assume a 'dysfunctional' state in need of correction or adaptation. The focus of therapy is primarily on the individual: less frequently, sometimes expediently, within a group setting.

Humanistic, or 'personal growth', psychotherapies assume the existence of a 'real self', distinct from the mechanistic mind-brain concepts of traditional psychological thought. These approaches assume that people define themselves, rather than are defined by others: change involves choice, rather than need. The personal goal is self-actualization: the person can 'be all that he or she can be'. There is no need to 'fit in': the person can be liberated from social conventions, rather than adjust and conform. This involves a developmental process: the person (ego) is enhanced. The person is not 'sick', nor defective, and so 'needs' no healing or repair. The focus of such therapies is commonly on people in groups.

Transpersonal psychotherapies assume the existence of a 'higher self' in which the person is defined by the Other: all such therapies are implicitly spiritual (see Assagioli, 1975). The person's motivation is to 'surrender' to forces which are cosmic, rather than personal and social: the personal goal is union with the infinite, salvation from the social constriction of human life. The process of such therapies involves a reduced emphasis on the ego, losing 'one's self' in pursuit of enlightenment. The typical focus of such 'therapies' is a supportive community, rather than the typical individual or group therapy sessions of traditional and humanistic sessions.

This method of distinguishing one therapy from another is complicated by the growing tendency of therapists to claim eclectic status. Psychoanalysts have tried to incorporate aspects of Zen, resulting in a 'traditional-transpersonal' graft (Fromm, 1987); behaviour therapists have incorporated aspects of Rogers' person-centred therapy (Barker, 1982) to become 'traditional-humanistic'. Some eclectic therapies highlight the value of behavioural assignments, within a humanistic framework, against a background of Buddhist philosophy: 'traditional-humanistic-transpersonal' (Reynolds, 1984). Even within specific 'movements', such as cognitive therapy, some practitioners, such as Meichenbaum (1977) are reductionist, by focusing specifically upon the mediating effect of 'self-talk' in facilitating the self-control of overt patterns of behaviour. Other cognitive therapists, such as Ellis (1984), claim to be 'doubly humanistic', and attempt: 'to help people maximize their individuality, freedom, self-interest and self-control' whilst at the same time helping them live 'in an involved, committed and selectively loving manner with other humans'. The observer might accept Ellis's philosophy as humanistic, but might be obliged to categorize his method as traditional. Ellis' technique emphasizes disputation and other overt attempts to encourage the person to relinquish one set of (dysfunctional) beliefs in order to acquire or employ, more adaptive strategies. In the sense that Ellis 'knows' what is right, and tries to convert people to that view, he is a 'normalist'. These few illustrations show the futility of trying to categorize specific therapies. From an ethical perspective it may be more appropriate to question the motives of the individual therapist: what is his purpose in manipulating one, or many, approaches in an effort to be helpful? Are all therapeutic technologies as Skinner (1973) observed, ethically neutral?

AIMS AND IMPLICATIONS

Given this range of theories what is the common aim of these attempts at resolving human misery? Are they concerned with changing the 'circumstances' of the person which act upon him/her, thereby producing the distress or disturbance represented by the 'complaint'? Or, are they concerned to 'help' the person influence the circumstances which might be seen to be influential, thereby producing some significant change witnessed, at least, within the person him/herself?

Different therapeutic aims provoke different implications for the therapist's role. Therapies which assume that the person is the 'object' of particular, non-specific, forms of 'influence', which produce the present problem of living, will acknowledge these (hypothetical) laws in the therapeutic relationship. Therapies which accept the person as a 'free agent', who acts in ways which affect the life experience, will build this construct into the working relationship. A distinction appears to exist between therapies which assume that people are 'determined' by circumstances largely outwith their control, and those which accept the fundamental 'freedom' of the person to act (see Chapter 7 by Jacqueline Atkinson).

Some therapies aim to 'modify' the way people live their lives, shaping or moulding the person, through their actions, to behave in specific ways. Such therapies appear to be based (overtly or covertly) upon manipulation: therapy involves handling the person with great interpersonal skill and may involve a clever manoeuvring of the person causing the person to act as the therapist wishes. Studies suggest that behaviour therapists are just as prone to show 'client'centred' interpersonal styles (Sloane *et al.*, (1975) as Carl Rogers himself was prone to use verbal reinforcement (Murray, 1956; Truax, 1966). Are the differences between therapies more theoretical than practical?

The extent to which different therapies 'oblige' the person to accept the therapist's view varies: some therapists may be more honest about their objectives than others. The central thesis of Ellis' 'Rational-Emotive-Therapy' is that emotional disturbances is caused by internal sentences repeated by the distressed person. In Ellis' view almost any emotional disturbance derives from an irrational belief which generates negative self-statements which, in turn, stimulate the negative emotional arousal. The therapeutic 'agenda' is very open: Ellis declares his view very early in the relationship. Not all therapists are quite so candid.

The setting of 'therapeutic goals' represents a further dimension. Do therapists allow people to determine their own 'goals', or do they attempt to 'engineer' the person towards making the 'right' choice? Lifton (1976) considered the problem of allegiance faced by many therapists. Did the therapist 'help' the person to adjust to social norms, or help the person to reach conclusions about the meaning of his or her own life? This conflict was heightened for Lifton in his work with traumatized Vietnam veterans: as a **professional** he needed to remain sufficiently detached to make a psychological evaluation; as a **person** he needed to acknowledge his own philosophical opposition to the war. Lifton's dilemma exemplifies the fallacious nature of so-called 'value-free' psychotherapy. 'Ethical' practice in psychotherapy may involve the recognition of the therapist's biases, and his or her potential for imposing them.

THE NEED FOR CHANGE

Proponents of various therapies might argue that their theory is 'theoretically valid', or supported by evidence of its value as a means of reducing psychological distress, modifying behaviour, or promoting 'growth' etc. Beliefs in the inherent 'value' of the therapies prompt consideration of the definition of 'problems' and the measurement of 'positive' change. Who defines the 'problem' and who decides that it has been resolved?

Many therapies are based upon simple beliefs about the genesis of problems of living and their resolution. Assertiveness training is advocated by therapists from a range of theoretical backgrounds, although it is rooted in behavioural theory. People who behave in a submissive manner, or who tend to dominate others, are often encouraged to become more 'assertive' by expressing their own thoughts and feelings in a direct and honest fashion whilst at the same time respecting the rights of other people (Lange and Jakubowski, 1976). But what, exactly, are 'our rights' and the 'rights of others'? Who, if not the therapist, provides these definitions? Given that many patterns of appropriate and inappropriate behaviour are culturally determined (if not also determined by individual value systems, such as religious conviction) there may be a danger in assuming that 'assertive behaviour' exists, any more than 'passivity or submissiveness' exist. Such patterns of behaviour are defined, largely, by others: a person acting in a particular way may be viewed as 'submissive'. The person, however, may view this situation differently, describing it as (for example) 'turning the other cheek'. Interpersonal behaviour, in this sense, is a relative, rather than fixed or measurable concept.

The identification of 'problems', and their possible resolution are culturally bound. A Christian experiencing interpersonal discord, might 'feel' like telling a partner what he or she thinks or feels, but may 'believe' that the 'right' response is to turn the other cheek. Such conflicts are an essential part of the formulation of the problem and are ignored at great cost.

The methods employed in various therapies also emphasize beliefs rooted in various theories. Some behavioural therapists might recommend the use of contingent electric shock to eliminate a dangerous pattern of behaviour, such as repeated vomiting (Lang and Melamed, 1969) or self-injury (Martin, 1975). Inflicting pain to change even such severe problem often generates strong feelings, and often serves as the basis of the myth of the clinical, calculating, cold-hearted behaviourist. Behavioural therapists might emphasize the necessity of such 'last resort' interventions, especially if non-aversive interventions have failed (see Chapter 9 by Chris Cullen). Is this issue limited only to behavioural therapies? What of the gestalt therapist, who encourages (obliges?) the person to face uncomfortable (painful) feelings which he or she has avoided for years? (Perls, 1976).

Similar experience of 'psychological anguish' is involved whenever people are obliged to confront loss, as in bereavement therapy, or to face phobic situations, as in flooding, or implosion. All psychoanalytic psychotherapy aims to lead people to realizations or 'insights', causing great anguish in the process: why else would people have 'repressed' them? Is such 'exposure' to the 'truth', cruel, heartless and unethical?

WHAT IS THE PROBLEM?

The value of psychotherapy depends on its effectiveness. In keeping with the medical diagnosis of pathology, problems of living are defined, commonly, in the early stages of therapist-patient contact. Although the idea that one specific therapy might be indicated for any one specific problem of living is not universally accepted, a general consensus exists that practitioners, if not recipients, want (or need) to know the utility of different therapies for different problems of living.

Do people, however, always seek help for what really 'ails' them? Is the problem 'submitted for therapy', always the real, or major, problem? Smail (1978) cited the example of a woman treated for 'sexual frigidity', in the context of an apparently happy marriage. After many months of therapy, the woman was offered sexual counselling which, after an initial enthusiasm, resulted in her 'admission' that the real problem was 'repulsion' for her husband, and an 'unexpressed' love for a neighbour. Smail observed that the presenting problem (frigidity) was 'symptomatic' of a relationship problem which the woman had 'resisted' acknowledging for many months. During this time she had diligently sought, and tried out, various 'solutions'. The 'cure' which had to be 'resisted', was the acknowledgement that she no longer loved her husband, with the accompanying threat to the happiness of her three children. Smail asserts that all therapists need to take seriously the expressed meaning of any problem a person brings to therapy. People may often describe how they engage in some problematic behaviour which they wish to cease: abusing drugs, being unfaithful to their partner, acting aggressively, and so on, whilst 'knowing' that they 'shouldn't' behave in this way. Smail suggests that the person's behaviour ('problem') always has meaning, whether or not he or she is aware of this. From an existential perspective, the person's behaviour has reasons which are 'chosen', rather than which act as inexorable forces upon the person.

The 'natural' aim of such a therapeutic analysis is to confront problems bodily, rather than through the largely intellectual exercise of introspection and emotional tinkering, with which many therapies are fraught. Knowing what the problem is, obtaining 'insight', provides no more than an outline of the possibilities of change. Smail (1978) argues that 'rumination' about problems will not help the person challenge his or her 'symptoms,' face fears, learn new social skills: for this end he or she needs 'courage' to fuel the bodily action necessary.

Such contemporary accounts of a desirable therapeutic practice reflect an age-old wisdom. Drawing on the practical philosophy of Zen writers. Watts (1968) described the 'Short Path', considered as a swift and steep ascent to *nirvana* for those who have the necessary courage . . . found in the 'Six Precepts' . . . :

No thought, no reflection, no analysis
No cultivation, no intention:
Let it settle itself.

An American 'Morita therapist' Reynolds (1984) paraphrases this Zen precept: 'Some say they can, some say they can't . . . let the action tell the tale.' This therapeutic attitude invites the person, albeit implicitly, to focus attention on the 'living' of life rather than upon an emotional experience, which may be no more than epiphenomenal — a 'secondary' experience which arises from the actual experience of living itself. In Western cultures, obsessed with emotion, such an attitude may provoke discomfort. Uncomfortable though such as idea may be, does that mean it is 'wrong'?

ADDRESSING THE PERSON

The person receiving psychotherapy is, traditionally, referred to as 'the patient': a convention applying to all people who receive medical intervention. Given that some psychotherapists have given much consideration to 'slips of the tongue' (or the 'true' meaning of verbal statements) the implications of use of the term 'patient' will be considered, as well as its popular alternative, client.

Usage of the term patient derives from the extension of the status of the person as a recipient of medical treatment even to situations where the physician's role is marginal, as in psychiatric care. The term presupposes a restricted view of normality and health: the person who is 'patient' lies outwith such normal limits and occupies, in effect, a pathological state. Critics of the stigmatizing nature of the label 'patient' suggest that the behaviour of the person may represent a reasonable response to a wholly unreasonable environment. Although the term 'patient' connotes suffering (as from a disease) the history of medical treatment suggests that patients have also been required to suffer 'unquestioningly' all manner of interventions, not all appropriate to their needs. Psychotherapists need to consider the power relationship between them and their 'patients'. Is the person required to exercise patience and 'sufferance', accepting any intervention considered necessary? If the person is not to be confined to this extent, why should any considerate therapist wish to re-define the person as 'patient'?

The term client, popularized by Rogers (1951), suggests that the person in therapy equates with the consumer of services in a capitalist economy. Outside of privately contracted therapy this is a gross distortion. People whose needs for psychotherapy are met within a health service provision are offered either whatever therapy is available locally, or will be 'referred' to the therapist considered most appropriate. The extent to which the person can exercise choice, selecting from some hypothetical menu of psychotherapeutic services, is unclear.

Although the person may not be 'purchasing' the service directly, he or she could, instead, be seen as paying indirectly through health insurance contributions. Does this signify, therefore, status as a client, or self-determining consumer? The options, are however, so limited as to deny the existence of any real choice. More importantly, some general psychotherapeutic service may be recommended: one which may have a questionable track record in terms of demonstrated efficacy in resolving the problems presented. This is akin to offering a householder with a plumbing, wiring, or building problem, the single option of servicing by the local jack-of-all-trades. How many householders would 'purchase' such services, in preference to servicing by a registered worker, proficient in one area? Equally, the services offered by a psychiatrist can be generic: unsupported by any specific therapeutic model and perhaps also lacking any identifiable expertise. People who need help with problems of living should expect a specialist service, rather than well-intentioned genericism.

The use of the term client in human services appears to derive more appropriately from the original Latin meaning *cliens*: a plebian under the patronage of a patron. In Roman times the client performed certain services: the patron, in return, protected the life and interests of the person. Although not identical, this appears to be a clear approximation to today's 'client' in the psychotherapeutic arena. Providing that the person fulfils certain requirements of the therapist — attending appointments, completing homework assignments, 'buying' the model of therapy on offer — the therapist agrees to act as her guide and mentor. The client-therapist relationship is a conditional one.

SPECIALIST OR NOVICE?

The person in therapy might well assume that his or her therapist not only believes in the therapy espoused, but is also a safe and competent practitioner. Not all practitioners will have had the benefit of training and some may try to become safe and competent by 'practising' on the person in therapy. Medical doctors undertaking training in psychiatry will 'practise' various forms of psychotherapy on their 'patients', as part of their

training. Are these patients advised about the novice status of their therapist? Wubbolding (1988) suggested that ethical practice in psychotherapy
and counselling should involve the practitioner giving the patient a statement of 'professional disclosure' describing the therapist's educational
background. In some states in the USA counsellors are required to give a
written statement containing their name, title, business address, telephone
number, formal education and areas of competence (see Wubbolding,
1988). Members of some psychotherapeutic 'movements' are bound by the
organization's Code of Practice: the British Association of Behavioural
Psychotherapy (BABP) expects its membership to abide by a carefully
defined code which aims to assure both quality and effectiveness. How
likely is it, however, that practitioners of all the therapies acknowledged
so far, will present the person with an objective evaluation of the efficacy of
the therapy on offer? As has already been noted considerable disagreement
exists as to what, exactly, needs to be evaluated.

POSSESSION OF THE PERSON

Many, though by no means all, therapies claim to represent a search for
either an 'improved' self, or even for the *true* self. Although the layperson's
notion that psychotherapy involves discovering the 'cause' of his or her
present distress is shared by few therapists themselves, psychodynamic
psychotherapies do aim to bring past experiences and present disabilities
into 'meaningful conjunction' (Walton, 1983). This view embraces a belief
that all clients have childhood traumas which they introduce to the therapy
situation, transferring these to the therapist, whom they perceive as similar
to the significant adult figures of their childhood. This view is greatly at
odds with other therapies which aim to establish more equal relation
between client and therapist, from the outset.

Another aspect of the concept is **transference neurosis**. This assumes
that people in therapy tell lies to protect themselves from the therapist.
The assumption here is that the therapist 'knows' the truth of the situation:
the 'patient' denies this reality, using defensive manoeuvres which Bion
(1970) saw as transparent 'lying'. Can the therapist ever really know the
person other than in an objective sense? This question raises the issue of
experiential and objective reality. When individuals who are patients talk
about themselves, they describe a reality which is 'experienced': a truth
which is 'felt'. The therapist, or indeed any outsider, sees an objective
reality: one which may be coloured by his or her own (subjective) experience, or may be defined within the parameters of the therapist's own
ideological perception of reality. When a blind person says 'I see what
you mean', he or she registers agreement based upon perception of some
internally-registered translation of a largely auditory objective reality. Convention dictates that this agreement is accepted, although this person is

even less likely to have 'seen' our meaning than would a sighted person. The sighting is metaphorical, as also is the concurrent understanding. But how firmly can it be established that the person has not grasped (firmly) the wrong end of the proverbial stick? What evidence exists to suggest that therapists have the capacity to 'see through' the transparent lying of people in therapy?

Some therapies attempt to integrate past and present experience; others have more mundane ambitions — the adjustment of patterns of living in pursuit of an improved 'quality of life'. Although the efficacy of traditional forms of therapy have proven difficult to assess, it is commonly assumed that therapies which do not manipulate past and present emotional experience are inferior. Forms of psychotherapy which aim, perhaps more realistically, at small-scale adjustment of styles of living, are dismissed as 'counselling'. Approaches which assume that patterns of living are determined by present, rather than past experience, such as the 'behaviour therapies', are dismissed as dealing only with symptom relief.

What is 'needed' here: a change in a style of behaviour (living life differently), or a change in perceived reality (thinking differently about life)? Many of the concerns debated within this chapter are largely of Western (Occidental) origin. Therapies which derive from a non-Western base, such as Morita's Zen-influenced psychotherapy (Reynolds, 1984), assume that the meaning of life is to be found in the living of it: emotional experience is largely tangential to the 'experiential reality' of behaviour.

HOLISTIC CARE AND REDUCTIONIST THERAPIES

Some mental health workers, such as social workers, and more recently psychiatric nurses, claim to express a specific interest in the 'whole person'. The relationship between ideas of 'holistic practice' and the care and treatment of the 'whole person' are not necessarily synonymous. Whether or not 'holism' is a valid concept is not at issue here. The concept does, however, raise a related issue in respect of the practice of 'holistic' therapies. Specifically, can practitioners who claim to practise 'holistic care' practise forms of therapy which are not 'holistic' and which, indeed, might be defined as focused, if not reductionist in nature? For example, can psychiatric nurses employ methods such as Ellis' Rational Emotive Therapy which (relative to some other forms of therapy) has a narrow view of the person's problems and the goals of therapy, while at the same time claiming to practice 'holistic' nursing care? The same question can be asked in relation to the practice of any 'reductionist' psychotherapy: that is, those which 'collapse' the person into a limited number of conceptual functional categories, such as psychoanalysis or conditioning therapies.

The validity of the 'holistic' approach is, however, not beyond question. Despite the sympathy evoked by the idea of dealing with the 'whole person' is this any more than a romantic fiction? It is possible to define the limits of the person, hypothetically, as a biological organism: in the terms derived from contemporary biological science. People can be trained and examined in a set of 'ideas' about the 'biological person' which derive from this knowledge-base. Although any professional is free to experiment with alternative formulations of the biological state, he or she is unlikely to be taken seriously, and may even be given short shrift by examining boards. In short, a consensus view exists as to 'what', exactly is a person, biologically speaking. Does any such consensus exist as to the idea of a 'whole person'. Such a concept embraces everything from molecular activity to the transpersonal self. Can any professional group ever establish whether or not an individual practitioner is using the term appropriately? Can any examining board ever 'test' the knowledge and skills base of a 'holistic (wholistic)' practitioner? And even if this were possible how do we know such a conceptual framework is more worthwhile than more reductionist models of care and treatment? More importantly, how might the person in therapy be helped to make such a comparative judgement?

From a psychotherapeutic perspective some 'holistic' models of therapy, for example the multimodal therapy of Lazarus (1976), have been proposed and practised. Is it ethical for nurses, social workers or any other professional group, to begin to define a holistic (multimodal) approach without acknowledging Lazarus' historical precedent? How much freedom should be extended to professionals who wish to re-invent the wheel? A related issue involves cost-effectiveness. Given that financial resources for mental health service delivery are finite, how tightly should available therapies conform to some 'gold standard' of efficacy? Should a mental health programme funded by taxpayers offer therapeutic services which are demonstrably 'ineffective', or 'effective but costly', or 'untestable' in terms of their assumed outcome variables?

HELPING AND THERAPY: A RAPPROCHEMENT

Although a behavioural approach to therapy is often equated with control at its worst, the role of 'control' in therapy can have positive connotations (see also Chapter 9 by Chris Cullen). Masters *et al.* (1987) described the behavioural approach as based upon the promotion of freedom, through the helping of the person in therapy they can gain more control over him/herself and ultimately over those aspects of the environment which exert an influence upon him or her. In their view this concept is rooted firmly in the behaviour 'therapist's' rejection of the traditional disease model of problems of living. Given that behaviour 'therapists' do not 'cure sickness' or 'eliminate illness', decisions about what is 'good' or 'bad' for the person in therapy become more complex. Citing Krasner, Masters and colleagues suggest that 'therapy' involves helping people 'learn how to control, influence or design their own environment'. Implicit in this is the 'value judgement that individual freedom is a desirable goal and that the more an individual is able to affect his/her environment, the greater is his freedom' (Krasner, 1976).

Traditionally, psychotherapy practised by male therapists on female patients has been open to abuse: much conventional psychotherapy is fraught with sexist problems bordering on misogyny. The unequal power relationship between male therapists and female clients has been viewed as a reflection of a social malaise and the distorted ideology of psychoanalysis itself (see Chesler, 1972; Showalter, 1987). The abuse of women by their therapist (Masson, 1989) may reflect no more than an exaggeration of the 'treatment' meted out to all 'patients'.

Although many therapists claim that therapy is a co-operative venture traditionally, at least, many therapists appeared to compete with the person, in a subtle power struggle. Although some therapies emphasize the collaboration of therapy-provider and therapy-recipient, in others, therapists often appear to be trying to outwit their subject: tricking the person into 'revealing', as Smail (1978) has observed, 'in an unguarded moment something about himself which can in any case only be of fleeting interest (p. 143)'. In Smail's view the psychotherapeutic 'techniques' which trick people into making such revelations are not only often wrongly applied, but are applied to the wrong end: there is no valid point in penetrating the 'guard' of the patient. Smail's assertion would, no doubt, be disputed by supporters of the psychodynamic method, but could they prove, in any demonstrable fashion, that his hypothesis was wrong? Alternatively, can they prove that their approach has any real point, beyond a momentary 'revelation'?

THE REJECTION OF THERAPY

Masson (1989) has argued vigorously for the rejection of all therapies on the grounds that psychotherapy, of all persuasions, is based upon a corrupt system: specifically, the witting manipulation of a gullible sufferer. Masson's critique is supported by verbatim transcripts and other 'admissions' from some of the leading figures in psychotherapy: Freud, Jung, Perls, and even Rogers, describe either largely inhuman treatment of distressed individuals or, in Freud's case, the manipulation of 'theory' to suit the popular tide of opinion (Masson, 1985). Masson appeared to err, however, by dismissing the theoretical formulations as a function of the individuals themselves. The critical *non sequitur* of his argument is that because the authors of various psychotherapeutic models behaved in a morally indefensible fashion, the theories themselves are immoral.

As psychiatry approaches the millenium it should be recognized that it cannot offer a satisfactory explanation of human distress simply by redefining the mind in terms of an increasingly elaborate description of the function of the brain (Healy, 1990). Even where evidence of physical, or physiological, disturbance can be offered as a partial explanation of disordered behaviour, the need for the person to analyze such disturbances and to 'reconstruct' his or her problems of living in meaningful terms, seems beyond question (at least on a human level). A truly 'objective' overview of psychotherapy research is a virtual impossibility, given the value-laden nature of most psychotherapeutic practice. The impartial view, such as it exists, seems to suggest that psychotherapies which focus upon the 'here and now' and which eschew the speculative, time-consuming interpretations of relationships between early experience and current life-problems, and other such untestable hypotheses, are a justifiable psychological currency. These relatively short, pragmatic, inquiring psychotherapeutic approaches are more likely to lead to the restitution of the 'patient' as the owner of a body of knowledge which might offer a genuinely personal explanation of life and how it might be lived. Justification for any school of psychotherapy which claims to 'know' people better than they know themselves appears to be more elusive. Given the preceding discussion, only therapies which can reassure recipients and critical professional observers that they aim to meet the individuals, human needs of the person can claim with any justification to hold the ethical ground.

CONCLUSIONS

The ethical correctness of psychotherapy *per se* is not at issue here. An idea cannot be criticized from a moral perspective. The appropriate focus for our concerns should be, the behaviour of psychotherapists. Identical forms of psychotherapy, in the theoretical sense, can be practised in ethical or unethical forms. An example of the unethical practice of psychotherapy was offered by Baron (1987). An English psychiatric day hospital, run as a 'therapeutic community', was closed after a series of internal inquiries stimulated by major staff-patient conflicts. Baron describes the events as examples of the 'tyranny of the therapeutic': the psychoanalytic model of treatment was used as an overt controlling force over every aspect of the patients' lives, whilst pretending to be libertarian. Baron's carefully-documented critique is a damning indictment of the covert power of psychiatric institutions, even when allegedly 'open' (Thompson, 1980). Baron does not, however, damn psychoanalysis: indeed, her report illustrates the abuse of people through the abuse of a therapeutic model. It remains to be shown, however, whether or not the model 'abused' in that setting had a greater potential to become a 'tyranical therapy'.

As the science of psychotherapy develops it needs to be evaluated critically from various standpoints: for example, comparative outcome efficacy and theoretical consistency. The art of psychotherapy, embraced by the various processes of the therapeutic relationship, needs critical examination from different perspectives. Of necessity, these might need to be more focused upon the experience of the recipient. How does the person judge the value of the service offered? Is the psychotherapist offering a genuine means of meeting personal needs, or has psychotherapy been subsumed within the highly controlling framework of psychiatry? Psychiatric expansionism ensures that other provinces are absorbed into the whole; research, behaviour therapy and 'pharmacotherapy' have been territorialized by psychiatry and psychiatrists for decades. These questions pivot around the practice of psychotherapy, the truth target for all our ethical deliberations. Psychotherapists, of all persuasions, need to recognize the bias which exits in any 'model' and the power to which all therapists have access. Recognition may help dismantle the 'objective' view of 'patients' which has bedevilled psychiatry, and construct more effective means of helping people understand their problems, and gain the necessary courage to act upon them.

REFERENCES

Assagioli, R. (1975) *Psychosynthesis: A Manual of Principles and Techniques*. Turnstone Books, London.
Banet, A. G. (1976) The goals of psychotherapy in Banet, A. G. (ed.) *Creative Psychotherapy: A Source Book* University Associates, La Jolla.
Barker, P. (1982) *Behaviour Therapy Nursing*. Croom Helm, London.
Baron, C. (1987) *Asylum to Anarchy*. Free Association Books, London.
Bion, W. R. (1970) *Attention and Interpretation*. Tavistock Publications, London.
Chesler, P. (1972) *Women and Madness*. Doubleday, Garden City.
Davison, G. C. and Neale, J. M. (1986) *Abnormal Psychology*, 4th ed. John Wiley, New York.
Edelson, M. (1977) Psychoanalysis as science: its boundary problems, special status, relations to other sciences and formalization. *Journal of Nervous and Mental Disease*. **165**, 1–28.
Ellis, A. (1984) Foreword in Dryden W. *Rational-Emotive Therapy; Fundamentals and Innovations* Croom Helm, London.
Erickson, E, (1976) Psychoanalysis and ethics: avowal and unavowal. *International Review of Psychoanalysis*. **3**, 409–15.
Fromm, E. (1987) *Psychoanalysis and Zen Buddhism* Unwin, London.
Healy, D, (1990) *The Suspended Revolution: Psychiatry and Psychotherapy Re-examined*. Faber and Faber, London.
Herink, R. (1980) *The Psychotherapy Handbook: The A to Z Guide to More than 250 Different Therapies in Use Today*. A Meridian Book, New American Library, New York.
Karle, H. (1989) Psychotherapy: method, magic or metaphor? *Changes*. **7** (1), 9–13.
Keith-Lucas, A. (1972) *Giving and Taking Help*. University of North Carolina, Chapel Hill.
Krasner, L. (1976) Behaviour modification: ethical issues and future trends. In Leitenberg H., (ed.) *Handbook of Behaviour Modification and Therapy*. Prentice-Hall, Englewood Cliffs, N.J.

Lang, P. J. and Melamed B. G. (1969) Avoidance conditioning therapy of an infant with chronic ruminative vomiting. *Journal of Abnormal Psychology*, **74** 1–8.

Lange, A. J. and Jakubowski, P. (1976) *Responsible Assertive Behaviour*. Research Press, Champaign, Illinois.

Lazarus, A. A. (1976) *Multimodal Behaviour Therapy*. Springer, New York.

Lifton, R. J. (1976) Advocacy and corruption in the healing professions. In Goldman N. L. and Segal D. R., (eds.) *The Social Psychology of Military Service*. Sage, CA. Beverly Hills.

Martin, R. (1975) *Legal Challenges to Behaviour Modification: Trends in Schools, Corrections and Mental Health*. Research Press, Champaign, Illinois.

Masson, J. M. (1985) *The Assault on Truth: Freud's Suppression of the Seduction Theory*. Penguin, Harmondsworth.

Masson, J. M. (1989) *Against Therapy*. Collins, London.

Masters, J. C., Burish, T. G., Hollon, S. D. and Rimm, D. C. (1987) *Behaviour Therapy: Techniques and Empirical Findings*, 3rd ed. Harcourt Brace Jovanovich, New York.

Meichenbaum, D. H. (1977) *Cognitive Behaviour Modification*. Plenum Press, New York.

Murray, E. J. (1956) A content analysis method for studying psychotherapy. *Psychological Monographs*, **70**, (13, Whole No. 420).

Perls, F. (1976) *The Gestalt Approach and Eyewitness to Therapy*. Bantam, New York.

Reynolds, D. (1984) *Playing Ball on Running Water*. Sheldon Press, London.

Rogers, C. R. (1951) *Client-Centred Therapy*. Houghton Mifflin, Boston.

Rorty, R. (1989) *Contingency Irony and Solidarity*. Cambridge University Press, Cambridge.

Showalter, E. (1987) *The Female Malady: women, madness and English culture 1830–1980*, Virago, London.

Skinner, B. F. (1973) *Beyond Freedom and Dignity*. Penguin, Harmondsworth.

Sloane, R. B., Staples F. R., Cirstol A. H., Yorkston N. J. and Whipple K. (1975) *Psychotherapy Versus Behaviour Therapy*. Harvard University Press, Cambridge, MA.

Smail, D. J. (1978) *Psychotherapy: A Personal Approach*. Dent, London.

Szasz, T. S. (1962) *The Myth of Mental Illness*. Secker and Warburg, London.

Szasz, T. S. (1978) *The Myth of Psychotherapy*. Anchor/Doubleday, New York.

Thomas, K. (1973) *Religion and the Decline of Magic*. Penguin, Harmondsworth.

Thompson, R. (1980) Psychotherapy: A refined form of hell on earth. *Nursing Mirror*, **150** (10), 33–5.

Truax, C. B. (1966) Reinforcement and nonreinforcement in Rogerian psychotherapy. *Journal of Abnormal Psychology*, **71**, 1–9.

Wachtel, P. (1977) *Psychoanalysis and Behaviour Therapy: Toward an Integration*, Basic Books, New York.

Walton, H. J. (1983) Individual psychotherapy. In Kendell, R. E. and Zeally, A. K. (eds.) *Companion to Psychiatric Studies*, 3rd ed. Churchill Livingston, Edinburgh.

Watts, A. (1968) *The Way of Zen*. Penguin, Harmondsworth.

Wubbolding, R .E. (1988) *Using Reality Therapy*. Harper and Row, New York.

Part Four

Chapter Eleven

Putting the service to rights

STEVE BALDWIN AND PHIL BARKER

EDITORS' INTRODUCTION

Much philosophical debate is abstract: an objective appraisal of the fundamentals of life, yet detached from ordinary experience. Although such
considerations have their place, mental health practitioners require more
immediate forms of enquiry. Without 'ordinary' examples of 'everyday'
ethical difficulties, practitioners could be excused for assuming that ethics
are a remote concept, and beyond their province. This could hardly be
further from the truth. The relative 'morality' of everyday actions, in
everyday settings, cuts across all professional boundaries. Although no
common 'code' of conduct exists to unite such disparate forces, such an
imperative is long overdue.

Although the delivery of any human service is now assumed to be a
stressful occupation, the basis of such stress is rarely attributed to the
ethical nature of activities. The need to address everyday, recurrent, ethical
conflicts remains unresolved: professionals need to set a firm ethical
agenda.

Putting the service to rights

Any consideration of ethical issues in mental health service delivery must
consider the rights of the person in care or treatment. To what extent are
those rights the same as those of other citizens; to what extent are they
different. If they are different, are those rights more, or less, protected. The
United Nations Declaration of Human Rights (UN, 1948) acknowledges the
need to respect the inherent dignity of all members of human race; the
rule makes no exceptions for sex, race, creed or social status. This declaration also acknowledges the individual's unalienable right to share the
benefits of scientific advancement: to enjoy the highest standards of physical and mental health possible, and freedom from medical treatment without informed consent. The Declaration reminds us, should we need
reminding, that the autonomy of women and men can be threatened,
especially in the health-care setting. Autonomy means preserving the

person's freedom of choice and right to self-determination. In some situations it may be difficult, if not impossible, to access the person's view: what the person wishes to be done. Such instances call for beneficence on the part of health care providers; making decisions which are truly in the best interests of that individual, rather than his or her family, community, state or even the health care workers themselves (Brody, 1989). In all instances, the person has a right to justice: equitable access to help or treatment, without unnecessary coercion or restraint. Helping people to exercise their access to these 'unalienable rights' will not always be easy for health care professionals: often people will decide that they do not wish access to the services on offer. As a result, professionals of all disciplines need to reflect on their relationship to the person in care, if not also to the system which supports that care. In a world of shifting values the need to establish the ethical agenda has never been more pronounced.

The following illustrations are distillations of actual experiences. Hopefully they may reflect the reader's own experience in covering similar ground — acting as ethical balance points upon which to consider some of the finer points of mental health morality. These short scenarios aim to illustrate dilemmas which elaborate some of the themes covered in previous chapters, or which stand alone, and remain unresolved.

THE ROOTS OF CARE

One evening a clinical psychologist visited a hostel for people with mental handicaps to discuss the progress of one of the residents with whom she was working. She overheard that a young woman, with whom she was not involved, was to have all her teeth removed the following day, due to an abscess on one of her teeth. The operation had been approved by the consultant psychiatrist, in consultation with the local dental hospital, although the young woman's general practitioner had not been informed.

The psychologist was concerned enough to wish to discuss this situation with her line manager: unfortunately he had gone to an evening meeting. She decided to talk to the unit administrator instead, taking care to translate the hostel incident into hypothetical person in a hypothetical service. The reality and urgency of the situation, however, came through and the administrator immediately contacted the hostel and instructed the staff to stop the admission to hospital. Although her name was not mentioned the psychologist thought that the hostel staff would be well aware of who had filed the complaint. She felt vindicated, however, when the administrator commented that she had acted 'most professionally'.

The hostel staff felt differently. The next day they were criticized sternly by their line manager for failing to stop the psychiatrist's unilateral action. The psychiatrist was incensed that his professional integrity should be so

challenged and talked in threatening tones about 'professional misconduct'. The dental surgeon, although he had not met the young woman,
supported the psychiatrist, further deepening the conflict.

In an effort to rescue the situation, the psychologist subsequently offered
to introduce a dental hygiene programme. The nursing team were
unhappy and unimpressed. Some of them felt that she had exposed them
to unnecessary criticism, and she felt distinctly unwelcome. Ironically, the
psychiatrist, who was the centre of both the decision and the resulting
conflict, shifted the responsibility (and guilt) on to the hostel staff.

On reflection the psychologist felt that she had made the right decision;
she would repeat her action in similar circumstances. Her colleagues,
however, were less supportive: the young woman was not her client, and
therefore not her responsibility; she was interfering, by setting herself up
as the independent 'advocate'; she had jeopardized staff morale by acting
impetuously, rather than 'sleeping on it'.

Themes

In a therapeutic community, such as a hostel or hospital ward, who has
responsibility for an individual who cannot speak for him/herself?

- How does a team, of different professional groups with differing experience and expertise, decide on the 'right' course of action for such an
  individual?

- What does a team do when faced with conflict and disagreement over
  such a decision?

- What kind of 'whistle blowing' procedure should exist in such a setting?

- What should any professional do when an 'irregularity' (whether minor
  or gross) is discovered?

- What is the appropriate behaviour for professionals who face conflicting
  situations, and who work in services which do not include advocacy
  systems?

Summary

Services for people are typically offered to groups: people with mental
handicaps, the elderly, people with chronic mental disorder, and so on.
This is largely an historical accident. If services were to be designed 'from
scratch' the individual would assume greater import. The group approach
to care can generate conflict within any service, especially where the needs
of one individual conflicts with another recipient of the same service. This
can be heightened where the needs of workers and 'consumers' conflict.
Where confusion about meeting individual needs exists an independent
advocacy system is required.

Similar tensions can exist whenever professionals from different disciplines are required to work together to provide a service. A possible solution to the inherent problems of teamwork may be to establish similar 'advocacy' services for professionals: an independent arbiter to provide truly independent advice. At present, the outcome of professional disagreements within teams may result in a systematic bias in favour of the discipline which is, professionally, the most dominant. Traditionally, medical staff have assumed such a dominant position; in other settings psychologists, for example, might try to assume the superior position.

Services need clear guidelines for use where conflict might arise. In any special care setting, supported by multidisciplinary teamwork, such conflict should be expected: if handled appropriately such conflict can be positive. Professionals who discover irregularities, or who suspect malpractice by design or default, need the security of team guidelines. Only if such guidelines were found to be inadequate, or impossible to implement, would third-party consultation prove necessary. It is apparent that professionals who work in services which continue to avoid, or reject, advocacy services, for consumer and provider alike, should expect conflict to be the rule rather than exception.

TAKING A STAND

A young psychologist took up post, along with two others, at a rural psychiatric hospital, one year after it had been the focus of a public enquiry. Despite some trepidation he was excited by the prospect: the expanding psychology department was committed not only to improving services to the residents and staff, but also to working towards organizational change within the hospital itself.

Two years later he felt only disillusionment. He realized that 'the problem' was more one of managerial obstruction, rather than clinical burnout. Malpractice among staff appeared to be condoned and gross misconduct passed without sanction. The system appeared to be geared more to staff convenience, rather than to the needs of the hospital population. Few, however, admitted to this state of affairs: those who did received little support. Prior to the public enquiry, two consultant psychiatrists had resigned over similar circumstances, and had vanished without trace.

Three years after his appointment the psychologist felt a similar obligation to resign: he could no longer be part of a 'care' system which systematically deprived people of their rights. It would be easy simply to move on: other posts were available, the field appeared open. However, he felt some responsibility to the people with whom he had worked. It would be irresponsible to leave without documenting this situation.

After several weeks he had produced a 5,000 word report, concluding with his personal opinion that the hospital should be closed. When it was published later in a national journal he agreed to appear on live television in a public debate. The hospital managers declined to appear, discrediting the report, saying that it was no more than a personal account. The next day the report was headline news. Within two days reporting stopped: the debate was over before it had really begun.

The psychologist had mixed feelings. He had received an opportunity to present his view of the issues through the media, but suspected that some form of censorship had turned the heat off the whole story. After an appearance on a live radio debate he concluded that the 'general public', although not disinterested, wanted to keep the hospital open, rather than risk exposure to 'crazy' or 'dangerous' people. His colleagues' responses were largely negative: slashed tyres and abusive threats on the telephone confirmed the level of feeling his public protest had aroused. A month later he resigned.

Themes

- To what extent is it appropriate for a professional to seek recourse to public debate in the media, over a professional issue?

- Is the professional contracted to provide services to clients only, or is he or she free to redefine the 'system' as the client?

- What are the limits to public disclosure of information about clients, workers or service systems, obtained whilst under contract?

- Should professionals who elect to be 'whistle blowers' expect personal and professional sanctions by colleagues within the system, whether peers or managers?

- Should professionals who criticize public institutions expect automatic public criticism?

- Should 'whistle blowers' speak out in public, or anonymously?

Summary

Professionals who elect to be 'whistle blowers' should expect negative criticism from colleagues, since their action inevitably threatens the stability of those remaining within the system. Professionals who seek third-party contacts as part of a critical debate risk professional isolation, as a price for any acclaim for their 'morally appropriate' or ethical behaviour. Where such action is considered, professionals should examine carefully their contractual obligations: how free are they to define the 'system' of care as 'the client'? Equally, there may well be limits to the amount, or nature, of information which can be disclosed to a third party, whether professional organization or media. Professionals who elect to 'speak out' in this fashion should recognize that this may make their former position untenable within the service. Most services do not appear to have reached the state of evolution whereby in-house critics, or other dissident voices, are rewarded for their contribution to the promotion of good practice. Until such time whistle blowers risk rejection and possible dismissal.

HOME AND AWAY

Joe was in his early fifties. He had lived at the large mental handicap hospital for almost all of his life. He had only a moderate degree of intellectual impairment, but was very nervous in company and struggled to hide a major speech impediment. He enjoyed good health: he was fit and strong, had worked in the hospital gardens and on the farm, and was a very good bowler, preferring the outdoor greens. He lived in a traditional ward with about 20 other men. He had an active social life. Most midweek nights he would go dancing, play bowls or go to a concert in the hospital. On Saturday he walked the mile long road to the nearest bus stop, often continuing a further five miles into the city if the weather was fine. After wandering around the shops he would head for one of the two football grounds where he had a stand pass. A quiet man leading a quiet life, Joe eased himself effortlessly from institutional to everyday life, and back again, attracting no special attention.

Almost overnight the climate of care for people with a mental handicap began to change in Joe's part of the country. One entrepreneur after another opened private homes for mentally and physically disabled adults, each finding the hospital a willing partner in supplying the 'residents'. Joe was an ideal choice: he presented no special care requirements; was quiet and amenable and, most importantly, would be unlikely to say 'No' to the invitation to move. Whether he actually wanted to go was less clear, but the staff at the hospital were unhappy about the proposal. The new facility was about 30 miles away, in a declining coastal resort. A small town with few amenities: the nearest football ground was his old 'home' territory. The home catered for about 25 residents, most of whom came from the hospital, but no-one with whom Joe had more than passing acquaintance.

Staff on the ward heard mixed reports about the new home and Joe's 'progress'. The consultant psychiatrist commented that this was community care: a smaller, more homelike setting, in the heart of a 'real' community. On a visit to the home one of the community nurses thought the residents were 'encouraged' to stay out most of the day, allowing the staff time to clean and prepare the evening meal. No special arrangements were made for activities: no special attempts to enable integration into the life of the small community. Joe was clearly an outsider looking in. He no longer bowled or went dancing. The same was true of the other residents: no longer institutionalized, life had become quieter than ever.

Themes

- Who should design the services for people who are disadvantaged, disabled or impaired?

- To what extent should people with handicaps be actively involved in the design of their own services?

- What conflicts occur when private sector competes with statutory sector to provide equivalent services?

- What conflicts occur for staff who have vested interests in both private and statutory sector services?

- When disagreements about specific options for clients occur, between direct-care staff and service managers, whose preferences should influence the outcome?

- Does physical presence in a locality or neighbourhood compensate for a restricted range of service options?

- Who will advocate for people who have been deinstitutionalized from hospitals?

Summary

Conflicts are bound to arise whenever staff are involved in multiple functions within the same service. Staff who provide direct services may not be able to be true advocates for people with whom they have an existing relationship. In such situations, conflicts of interest will imbalance their views: inevitably, their own needs as workers will dominate. Where clients have been omitted from the planning and development of their service, special efforts need to be made to encourage their active participation.

To avoid such conflicts of interest, staff need to distinguish the different functions of the service. This may be particularly important with regard to funding. New service designs, such as service brokerage, may be needed to achieve this. Disagreements between service managers may require 'third party' assistance, such as advocacy or arbitration, if the client's rights are not to be prejudiced. Deinstitutionalization will not, of itself, guarantee quality of life. Indeed, quality may be reduced if an equivalent range of service are not available, or if pre-existing relationships are not maintained. The service's 'march of progress' may well mask retrogression for the clients themselves.

WHO IS THE CLIENT?

Hassan and his brothers came to England in the mid 1960s. They worked in the textile industry at first then, after building some capital, opened a small store, selling fabrics. The business prospered and the brothers owned several properties and a chain of shops within the next 15 years. Hassan had had a normal childhood, with no major health problems. In his late twenties, however, he began to have mood swings, becoming suspicious of his brothers, who he accused of trying to cheat him. As the family business prospered, Hassan went into decline. His two brothers finally had to replace him when he was admitted to the local psychiatric hospital with a diagnosis of schizophrenia.

Hassan spent more than half of the next five years in hospital. He achieved some sort of stability with long-acting major tranquillizers and the support of the community psychiatric nursing service. Attending a local work centre each day he learned simple office skills each morning and participated in various social activities each afternoon. His mood was mainly 'blunted': he said little and continued to appear somewhat suspicious of the others at the centre. One afternoon in mid Summer, without warning, Hassan climbed on to the roof of the day care centre and threw himself from the four-storey building. He survived, but not without incurring crippling injuries. Unable to walk and with a speech impediment Hassan experienced frustrations with everyday life which further complicated his mental disorder.

The professional input to Hassan's care swelled, of necessity, following his discharge from hospital after his suicide attempt. Visits by the consultant psychiatrist, a social worker and occupational therapist were added to the continued presence of the CPN. An educational psychologist also joined the 'team' when one of Hassan's two children, by his young English wife (whom he had married just prior to his breakdown), showed some 'school avoidance'.

Two years after his discharge from hospital, Hassan's wife complained to her general practitioner of vague abdominal symptoms. When all tests proved negative she was referred to a psychiatrist, who referred her to a behavioural psychotherapist for 'relaxation'. Hassan's wife was tense, of this the therapist had no doubt. Relaxation appeared to be the least of her immediate needs. The assessment interview had produced a flood of tears, much suicidal ideation and a detailed catalogue of the misery which she had, and continued to experience with Hassan. She was uncertain of her feelings for her husband who was not the man she had married. She was caught between two cultures, feeling she belonged neither to the English society of her parents, nor the Moslem world of Hassan and his family. At first the therapist offered only a 'listening ear', later encouraging her to review her immediate problems, experimenting with possible solutions. As the therapeutic relationship deepened the 'unspoken desire' to escape from Hassan and to begin life afresh grew stronger.

The therapist's hypothesis was all the more unnerving since the therapeutic team, focused on Hassan, were oblivious to his wife's predicament. She was part of Hassan's 'social support system', rather than someone with her own needs. The dilemma sharpened for the therapist as her relationship with Hassan's wife deepened. She was uncertain of where her responsibilities lay: should she support Hassan's wife, helping her to solve her own life problems, knowing that it might lead to a withdrawal of support for Hassan himself? Or should she try to help his wife 'cope' better, provide her with the relaxation training first recommended, helping her mask her deeper anxieties, to remain a support to her husband? The dilemma would yield a bad outcome for one of the partners. Which was it to be? Who was the client?

THEMES

– What are the ethical problems inherent in providing psychiatric services for people who have pyschosocial problems, rather than obvious disorders or illnesses?

– When contact with one person leads to the identification of new, and different, needs of other persons, how is this best resolved by the professional?

– To what extent can one therapist 'cross boundaries', redefining the person's problem in terms of some significant other, such as spouse or family?

– At what point do cultural differences impede therapeutic progress, and how should professionals respond to this impasse?

– Can one professional represent the needs of more than one person in any one situation?

Summary

Professionals who have achieved competence in specific areas need to recognize the limits of their expertise and should be prepared to 'refer on' to other therapists. Equally, therapists should be aware that the actions of colleagues may be prejudicial to the needs of their client. Where such conflict exists professionals should try to negotiate a credible alternative, avoiding undermining their own position, or that of colleagues.

Contact with clients who have multiple needs, or with those with partners, families or carers with rival needs, require a special kind of contract between therapist and client. Therapists need to recognize that referral to help an individual differs markedly from a referral to 'treat' a family system. Where the family system, or the care being offered to part of that family system, conflicts with the service to one individual, that conflict must be aired. Failure to do so may lead to the suffocation of individual needs.

ADDING INSULT TO INJURY

Psychology technicians can have a dull routine: Jenny, who had just joined two other technicians in a small clinical psychology service, found the job an exciting challenge. She had lots of supervision and felt she was learning much. Her project took her all over the hospital and she often collected data in the evenings and weekends when the wards were quieter. One evening, a few months into the project, she headed for one of the wards to carry out some observations. Passing the adjoining ward she caught sight of one of the nursing assistants helping an older woman into bed. Jenny saw the nurse lean forward and strike the woman on the back of the hand with a hairbrush. Her eyes had not deceived her: she saw the incident, as though in a scene from a film, she reflected later. Jenny continued into the adjacent ward, as though nothing had happened, completed her recordings and went home.

Jenny mulled over the incident that night. There were several things she could have done: mentioned it to the nurse herself, spoken to the ward sister or the staff nurse. She knew them all well: indeed, she was on good terms with them. It troubled her that she had taken none of these options. She could also have spoken to her Head of Department who was strong on ethical issues. He might have put the incident into some sort of perspective. Or, she could have discussed it with the other technicians, or the psychologists she knew locally. There were so many options, as far as clarifying how she felt, deciding on how best to act, and yet she did nothing. The fact that, as a mere technician there were no obvious costs involved in 'speaking out', confused her even further. It would have been so easy to share and yet she did nothing.

She reflected on the incident a year or so later: it was a singular event which she never saw repeated. The hospital had a good reputation, so she wasn't altogether surprised. But she still found it hard to explain why she had failed to take any action. There was no potential penalty for her. Since she wasn't in training, or part of any hierarchy, no real sanctions could have been imposed. She could even have drawn attention to the incident with an anonymous comment. But still she had said nothing.

She often told herself that it was not a serious incident. This was unconvincing: what was serious was her ignorance of the event. At the very least she should have clarified, openly, what had taken place. Assaults on people were always serious. She vowed that in future she would always act at whatever cost to herself.

Themes

– What ethical dilemmas confront professionals who choose not to act in situations where action is appropriate?

- To what extent are decisions about action (or inaction) personal, rather than professional choices?

- Can 'acceptable levels' of physical or psychological damage ever exist for people in care?

- Should professionals view any incident of neglect, harm, abuse or damage, as an automatic indicator of the need to take positive action?

Summary

All workers in human services will encounter, at some time, incidents which raise ethical questions about the quality of treatment of those in care. Workers are likely to identify discrepancies between what should happen and what actually happens: this may be due to inadequate training or insufficient managerial guidance. The decision to take action, or not, over such discrepancies will, ultimately, be a personal decision. This may involve an appraisal of the potential cost, or benefits likely to be incurred, at a professional or personal level.

There exists a need for services to develop explicit contractual requirements which encourage workers to 'speak out' without fear of recriminations. Other service systems, such as airlines, have achieved this through anonymous positive reporting of incidents. These do not incur any costs to the individual, and generate important information from which managers can improve the quality of the service. Workers who find it difficult to assess the seriousness of observed 'deficiencies' should consider their feelings were the event to happen to them, or perhaps more importantly, to someone close to them. Each failure to act threatens a gradual erosion of personal ethical standards.

LIMITED COMPANY

The mental handicap assessment unit was staffed by a very positive multi-disciplinary team, all of whom were committed to a learning model. Bob was the first undergraduate student nurse to be placed at the centre, and he was excited about the experience which lay ahead.

Twelve young people attended the centre, each of whom was either being assessed or receiving some form of special education or therapy. Derek was a big, strong 15-year-old who was described as being 'out of control'. The Unit psychologist had developed a programme using the behavioural technique of time out, but it was clear to Bob that the approach wasn't working. Although no expert, Bob had studied operant theory as part of his course, having read more out of his own interest. The psychologist, however, seemed to have a quite different concept of time out from the model Bob had studied and read about.

There were several problems which, Bob felt, would have been obvious even to someone not versed in behavioural theory. Derek's programme involved withdrawing him from social situations if his behaviour was inappropriate. What exactly 'inappropriate behaviour' involved, however, was never defined. With more than eight staff involved, this led to many interpretations. Bob observed him being sent into time-out for 'not being polite', for being disruptive, and even for not eating his greens at lunchtime. Bob thought that perhaps the staff had been using the programme for so long, about three months, that they had lost sight of their objectives and any real objectivity.

Bob plotted the number of times Derek went into time out and found that it was steadily increasing, week by week. In Bob's second week at the Unit, Derek spent over two hours out of the five-hour day, in time out; more importantly, he seemed to 'ask' to be put into time out, and then would get involved in a furious struggle with staff, as they dragged him to the time out room at the other end of the building. The room itself seemed inappropriate: there was no observation point, and staff would often be showered in urine or spit as they opened the door, to let him out. Ironically, this outcome fitted in with the psychologist's rule that Derek be let out after ten minutes had elapsed, no matter what he was doing. More often than not he was as disturbed coming out, as when he went in.

Bob plucked up the courage to talk to the psychologist about the programme after five weeks. He didn't want to appear as a smart-alec, but he felt that Derek was not being handled properly. The programme hadn't even been explained to Derek on the grounds that he wouldn't understand. Bob was apprehensive: he knew that his placement report would be influenced by the whole team view, but he felt this nettle need to be grasped.

The psychologist didn't appear to take him seriously, making a wry comment about Bob having been 'reading up on the literature'. Bob argued that Derek's behaviour was getting worse: that he even appeared to enjoy going into time out. (Derek had said the previous week that he had 'fun with the nurses . . . more fun than in the Centre'). The psychologist was unmoved. He didn't argue, he was simply unmoved. Bob found some support among the rest of the team, but this evaporated when he brought up the issue at the weekly team meeting. The psychologist was the expert: Bob was a student, undergraduate or not.

Finally, he summarized the whole scenario in a short report, even predicting, in line with psychological thinking, the likely outcome of the programme. The unit sister showed this to the consultant psychiatrist. Although he showed some interest, clearly he had no real knowledge of behavioural analysis and, ultimately, he simply reprimanded the psychologist for allowing a student to create so much trouble in the Unit. From then on Bob's experience at the Unit went into decline: he felt himself simply waiting to be released from his own 'time out'.

At the end of his 13-week placement the psychologist apologized for the 'hard line' he had taken. He had to be careful; his future prospects were at risk. Bob left the Unit wondering who would act, honestly, in Derek's interests, rather than simply protecting their cwn.

Themes

– To what extent should any unqualified worker challenge the decisions of qualified professionals?

– What options remain for the worker who has exhausted all the legitimate lines of enquiry?

– Can a worker, who has a paid relationship with a person, also act as that person's advocate in the professional setting?

– What conflicts exist for staff whose progress depends on positive reports from line managers, with whom they may come into conflict?

– To what extent do professional codes of practice protect the rights of the person, and safeguard professionals using them to protect the people in their care?

Summary

Unqualified workers are a vulnerable group: their future employment in the service may be threatened if they challenge the authority of the qualified staff. Their unqualified status may also deprive them of any credibility, in the eyes of professional colleagues: this may obstruct them from taking action on incidents which raise ethical problems. It should not be assumed, however, that professional background or training is the most important factor in determining whether or not individuals can make appropriate comment on services or procedures. Although absence of qualifications alone does not disqualify workers from taking ethical action to remedy some deficiency, it may influence how they proceed.

Action by an individual will, inevitably, be viewed as a threat to the cohesion of the care system. Attempts to influence other workers or to enlist their support may be seen as a further threat, undermining the values of the system. All workers in any human service have responsibilities towards clients which extend beyond their job descriptions and professional guidelines. Professionals need to consider whether or not they are 'aiding and abetting' the abuse of clients, should they fail to challenge what they consider to be inappropriate models of care. In this sense, their view of the rights of people in care, should be no different from their view of their own rights, or those of the average citizen.

A SHOCK TO THE SYSTEM

Carol was a 15-year-old who had been admitted to a child psychiatric unit with an 'eating disorder'. Three months after admission she was given a course of six ECT's. An occupational therapist had been involved with Carol from her admission, working closely and intensively with her in building a trusting, confiding relationship. The occupational therapist was concerned about the use of ECT with a minor and made her anxieties known to the Unit team, to no avail. Still concerned, she discussed this with a clinical psychologist colleague, who confirmed her suspicions that ECT was not a recommended treatment for either eating disorders or minors.

Although the ECT had been suspended, the alternatives offered by the medical and nursing team appeared equally reductionist: a contingency management programme built around confinement to the ward. No interest appeared to be shown in dealing with the girl's specific difficulties in a personal, understanding manner.

Although he was not involved directly, the clinical psychologist was concerned that the treatment being offered was neither right nor fitting. He discussed his concerns with his line manager who was indifferent: he was not involved, it was none of his business. Unsatisfied, the psychologist took his concerns to the general manager who, although sympathetic, thought that the issue was not sufficient to challenge the authority of the medical team. Aware that his lack of direct involvement might well mean that he could not comment, the psychologist decided to take professional advice. His Code of Conduct was quite clear: he had an obligation to advocate on the girl's behalf if he thought that her treatment was inappropriate, inadequate, or in any way prejudicial to her wellbeing.

This finding posed some problems: how, exactly, could he act? Since he was not involved with their daughter, he decided to offer his services to the parents. Accompanied by the occupational therapist he outlined, to Carol and her parents, what options were available in terms of psychotherapy and counselling. The parents decided to withdraw their daughter from the Unit, and she enrolled in individual therapy with the psychologist. After five months she was discharged from therapy and returned to school. This was not, however, the end of the affair for the psychologist. Due to pressure from the medical staff the general manager threatened him with dismissal, warning also that the incident could have a negative effect on his career prospects. It had been brought to his attention that the psychologist was preparing a case study for publication; the manager issued a stern warning that such action might be libellous.

For the psychologist the 'case' was closed, but the issues arising from it were not. He needed to decide whether or not to publish what was an important addition to the literature on ECT and the psychological treatment of children. What was more important, his career prospects or the protection of an individual?

Themes

– Are some interventions, treatments, therapies, always inappropriate, or merely inappropriate in some situations?

– How may one professional legitimately challenge the decisions of another?

– What legal rights exist for people who are multiply disadvantaged and at risk?

– Where conflict between two professionals from the same discipline exists, how may this be resolved?

– What consequences exist for professionals who decide to act as an advocate, but come into conflict with their managers in the process?

Summary

All providers of mental health services will encounter situations which they deem to be intolerable or unacceptable. Their frequency will vary: for people at the 'cutting edge' of service delivery, this may well be a daily occurrence. Professionals frequently find that their training has not prepared them to face the kind of ethical dilemmas which they ultimately experience. Many workers have to draw upon personal resources where the necessary guidance is not available. Paradoxically, professionals who elect to follow their codes of conduct, as a guide to their own personal values, may find themselves alienated as a result. Although codes of conduct may be written to protect both the consumer and the provider, professionals should not always expect that their observance will attract popularity.

Inevitably, some highly qualified workers will fail to act because they perceive the risks to themselves as too costly. If the rights of the individual are to be protected, however, professionals who find themselves in disagreement with colleagues, however different in status, should challenge their judgements. Although the establishment of what is 'right' or 'fitting' may be difficult, professionals should never assume that good practice can be taken for granted.

Workers are accountable to their clients, their colleagues, employers and to society. Each worker has a responsibility to determine where his or her ultimate responsibility rests. Within these constraints, many workers will decide that they are, ultimately, responsible to themselves, and will operate according to a personal ethical code.

CONCLUSIONS

Consideration of these scenarios suggests that many professionals discover the ethical 'cut off' in the field of practice. How many consider, in advance, what should be the limits to which they, or their clients, should be compromised?

How many professional disciplines are prepared, from the outset of their professional training, to respect the United Nations Declaration of Human Rights? Many workers might be forgiven if they confessed to not knowing the Declaration, far less using it in their everyday work.

Ethics are an everyday concept. Ethics are not, or should not, be some form of navel-gazing, or observation of the care setting from a remote vantage point. Raising questions about 'ethical issues' can, too often, be interpreted negatively as 'trouble-making'. In many situations the 'trouble' already exists, in the form of inadequate or inappropriate service. The emphasis of traditional ethical debates upon 'major' issues, such as abortion, euthanasia and sterilization, may have misled many workers into thinking that ethics are not the 'stuff' of everyday life. For mental health workers ethics should underpin each and every action: no issue, however small, should be considered 'beneath' the ethical debate.

RECOMMENDED READING

Ashley, J. A. (1976) *Hospitals, Paternalism and the Role of the Nurse.* Teachers College Press, New York.

Barker, P. (1980) Ethics, nursing and behaviour modification. *Nursing Times,* **76** (22), 976–8.

Barker, P. and Baldwin S. (1990) Shock story: the use of ECT for children and adolescents. *Nursing Times,* **86**, (8), 52–55.

Beardshaw, V. (1981) *Conscientious Objectors at Work.* Social Audit, London.

Bernzweig, E. P. (1980) When in doubt — speak out. *American Journal of Nursing,* **80**, 1175–1176.

Brody, E. E. (1989) New horizons for liason psychiatry: Biomedical Technologies and human rights. *American Journal of Psychiatry,* **146**, (3), 293–295.

Culver, C. M., Ferrell R. B. and Green R. M. (1980) ECT and the special problems of informed consent. *American Journal of Psychiatry,* **39**, 951–958.

Dimond, B. (1987) Your disobedient servant. *Nursing Times,* **83**, (4), 28 January, 28–31.

Gaylin, W. (1982) The 'competence' of children. *Journal of the American Academy of Child Psychiatry,* **21**, 153–162.

Kurtines, W. M. (1986) Moral behaviour as rule governed behaviour: person and situation effects on moral decision-making. *Journal of Personality and Social Psychology,* **50**, (4), 784–791.

Morris, P. (1987) Prisoners of conscience. *Nursing Times,* **83**, (20), 16–18.

Olesen, V. L. (1989) Caregiving, ethical and informal: emerging challenges in the sociology of health and illness. *Journal of Health and Social Behaviour.* **30**, 1–10.

Pyne, R. (1987) A duty to shout. *Nursing Times,* **83**, (42), 30–31.

Sclafani, M. (1986) Violence and behaviour control. *Journal of Psychosocial Nursing,* **24** (11), 8–13.

Sherlock, R. (1986) My brother's keeper? Mental health policy and the new psychiatry. In Kentsmith, D. K., Salladay, S. A. and Miya, P. A. (eds.) *Ethics in Mental Health Practice*. Grune and Stratton, New York.

Silverman, W. A. (1989) The myth of informed consent: in daily practice and clinical trials. *Journal of Medical Ethics*, **15**, 6–11.

Szasz, T. (1989) Psychiatric justice. *British Journal of Psychiatry*, **154**, 864–869.

United Nations General Assembly Committee on Human Rights (1977) *Report of the Human Rights Committee of the United Nations General Assembly*, United Nations, New York.

Vousden, M. (1987) End of an affair. *Nursing Times*, **83**, (20), 18–19.

Wilson-Barnet, J. (1989) Limited autonomy and partnership: professional relationships in health care. *Journal of Medical Ethics*, **15**, 12–16.

Chapter Twelve

In search of ethical parameters

PHIL BARKER AND STEVE BALDWIN

INTRODUCTION

The ethical issues raised in the preceding chapters reflect, to a great extent, the authors' personal ethical philosophies. It is fitting, therefore, that the editors conclude with a brief exposition of their ethical philosophy. The recommendations which follow reflect our view of 'good behaviour' in human services. These reflect the guiding principles which serve as the ethical parameters to our work: they are appropriate to all client groups — for example, people with learning difficulties or mental handicap, young people, older people, people with mental or physical disability.

These recommendations cut across all professional disciplines. Equally, they may be of relevance to groups and agencies offering non-statutory services to people with problems of living. For convenience, we use the term 'problems of living' to refer to any difficulty people experience, whether influenced by physical, psychological or social factors, or by any combination of these influences.

The recommendations refer in every case to the service offered to 'the person': we regard the person, or individual, as primary; the needs of families, society or service providers, are of secondary consideration and, therefore, are not addressed here.

ETHICAL SERVICE DESIGN PRINCIPLES

Advocacy

– Every person receiving a service should have access from the point of entry to the support of an **independent** advocate.

– Service providers should acknowledge that professionals **cannot**, indeed should not, be asked to act as the advocate for the person with whom they have a professional relationship.

– Service providers need to recognize that although they may be responsible for funding the advocacy service, they are not responsible for its direction.

– Where advocacy is provided as part of a professional service, advocates should be expected to meet agreed standards of competence.

Access

– Appropriate services should be offered to the person **irrespective** of age, sex, colour, creed, culture, sexual or political orientation.

– The person with **any** special need, should have free access to all other (generic) services, in addition to the provision of any special needs service.

– All people with problems of living should have free access to any service which they consider potentially appropriate to their needs.

– Where equitable access does not exist, all professionals should assume the responsibility of ensuring that the extra support necessary is provided.

– The person or advocate should have the right of access to all personal records.

Assessment

– For ethical service delivery, comprehensive, individualized assessment should be seen as the primary objective.

– The process of assessment should involve the person, and where appropriate, the advocate.

– All professionals should acknowledge that assessment is done **with**, rather than to, the person and/or the advocate.

– All assessment should aim to identify the **individual** needs of the person, as distinct from the needs of any significant other.

Aims

– All services should treat people with dignity and respect, confirming their inherent worth at all times.

– All services should be offered unconditionally.

– The overall aim of any service should promote the positive development of the person, rather than the removal of negative characteristics.

– The end-point of treatment, or intervention, should be defined, consistent with the person's needs.

– The process of treatment or intervention, and all the stages therein (means), should be consistent with the overall aim (end).

– Professionals should define clearly, and record accurately, their discussion with the person, or advocate, which involves setting aims or objectives.

- Professionals should negotiate to monitor the process of service delivery, with full consent and co-operation of the person or the advocate.

Consent

- Professionals should recognize only **valid** consent: that which is given freely, without coercion, and supported by knowledge of the costs and benefits of any intervention or treatment.

- Where valid consent cannot be obtained, professionals should firstly recognize only the 'third-party' consent of the person's advocate.

- Where such 'third-party' consent cannot be obtained, professionals should obtain independent advice, from someone not directly involved with the person.

- Where consent cannot be obtained from any of the above sources, professionals are obliged to evaluate the possible outcomes of any intervention (or non-intervention) on behalf of the person, and act accordingly.

Methods of intervention or treatment

- Professionals should recognize the primary need to offer the person a range of options.

- Consistent with the overall aim, all interventions should promote the positive development of the person, rather than emphasize the removal of negative characteristics.

- The options on offer should be explained to the person in non-technical language, including information about possible costs, benefits and ultimate outcomes.

- Professionals should recognize that 'costs' to the person can involve physical, financial, emotional and time consequences; these considerations should be discussed fully with the person or the advocate.

- The person should be free to discontinue with the service at any time, without cost.

- The treatment or intervention options should be drawn from quality methods which are both cost-effective and appropriate to the person's needs.

- Where alternative (unproven or non-established) methods are offered, these should represent the least restrictive option.

- Restrictive, aversive or coercive methods should be used only with the valid consent of the person or the advocate, providing that all other appropriate non-restrictive, non-aversive and non-coercive methods have been exhausted.

Evaluation

- The process of service delivery should be monitored systematically from outset to outcome.

- Professionals have an obligation to use reliable and valid methods of assessment to identify needs and measure outcomes.

- Professionals have an obligation to use the evaluation to amend or suspend any intervention when necessary.

- The person or the advocate should be actively involved in the process of evaluation.

Accountability and responsibility

- Professionals should recognize that their primary accountability is to the person at all times.

- Professionals should operate only within the bounds of their competence.

- When professionals have reached the limits of their competence they should enlist the support of colleagues with alternative skills or knowledge.

- Professionals should refer to alternative agencies when appropriate.

- Professionals should recognize a wider responsibility to their colleagues, and other people receiving the service.

Index